Writing HERSTORY

———— A MEMOIR ————
FEATURING 18 WOMEN & HERSTORY

Writing HERstory

2023 YGTMedia Co. Press Trade Paperback Edition.
Copyright © 2023 Ashley Lougheed

All Rights Reserved. No part of this book can be scanned, distributed, or copied without permission. This book or any portion thereof may not be reproduced or used in any manner whatsoever without the express written permission of the publisher at publishing@ygtmedia.co—except for the use of brief quotations in a book review.

The author has made every effort to ensure the accuracy of the information within this book was correct at time of publication. The author does not assume and hereby disclaims any liability to any party for any loss, damage, or disruption caused by errors or omissions, whether such errors or omissions result from accident, negligence, or any other cause. Some names and identifying details have been changed to protect the privacy of those discussed.

The publisher is not responsible for websites (or their content) that are not owned by the publisher.

Published in Canada, for Global Distribution by YGTMedia Co.
www.ygtmedia.co
For more information email: publishing@ygtmedia.co

ISBN trade paperback: 978-1-998754-35-9
ISBN hardback: 978-1-998754-37-3
eBook: 978-1-998754-42-7

To order additional copies of this book:
publishing@ygtmedia.co

AUTHOR'S NOTE:
The content of this book is based on my interpretation of events to the best of my recollection. My stories are not meant to challenge or judge anyone.

Writing HERSTORY

―――― A MEMOIR ――――
FEATURING 18 WOMEN & HERSTORY

Ashley Lougheed

Lots of Love,
Ashley xo

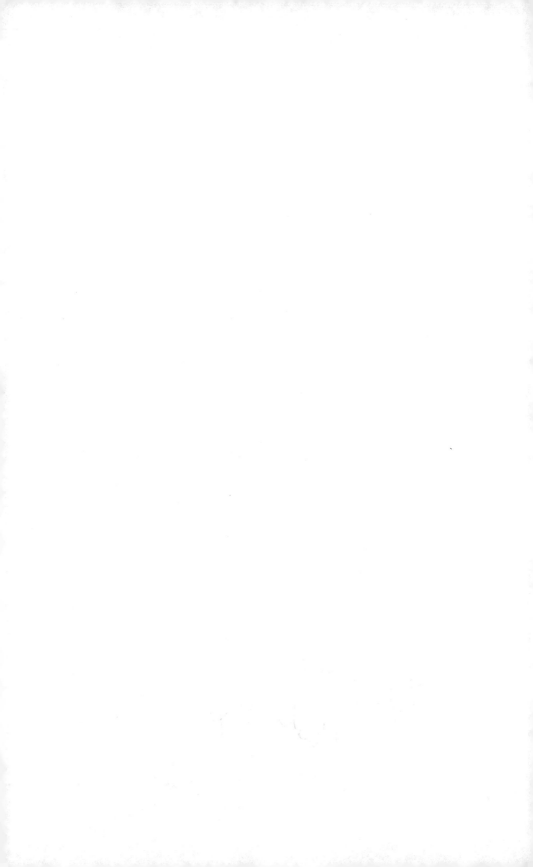

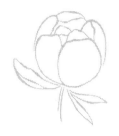

Trigger Warning:

Sexual assault, suicidal ideation and attempted suicide, body dysmorphia, disordered eating, parental abuse, emotional abuse, alcoholism, grief, death

Dedication:

To my eight-year-old self and my eighty-year-old self.
You are HER. My hope is that you always find
your power in your voice and bravery in each step
toward your life's purpose. You were born with self-worth:
an inner confidence, your definition of success, and the
ability to love yourself and others.

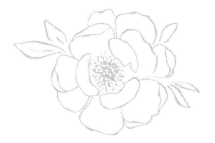

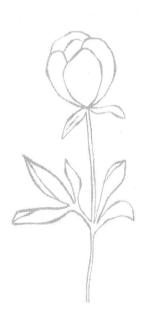

Table of Contents

Prologue 01

Introduction 04

Chapter 1: Birth of a Girl 17

Chapter 2: The Search for Identity 29

Chapter 3: It's a Girl Thing 49

Chapter 4: Being Labeled and the Power
of Knowledge 73

Chapter 5: Friendship, Love, and Romance 91

Chapter 6: Transitions and Choices 111

Chapter 7: Motherhood 133

Chapter 8: Relationship Challenges
and Finding Grit 149

Chapter 9: Leaning on Sisters; Believing in Self 167

Chapter 10: Loss and Heartache 187

Chapter 11: Girl Time 207

Conclusion 221

Acknowledgments 227

Resources 234

References and Works Cited 235

Prologue

I was flying through the air, the ground only seconds away. I knew before I hit that Duke, my ever-faithful companion, had stopped short of taking the leap. On impact, the ground, hard and unforgiving, took my breath away. Shaken and bruised, I wanted to lie there forever.

I wasn't involved in extracurricular sports throughout my school years. My interests were in dance and horseback riding. Dance was a way for me to move my body and fully express myself. I loved listening to the rhythm and beat and then moving in a way that matched them. Dance became my version of being a part of a team. Horseback riding, though, that was different. It was just me and my horse, Duke.

  I felt at ease in the barn with the horses and barn cats and Jenny, my riding instructor and role model. Jenny's first lesson was all about grooming Duke's hooves, brushing him, and preparing him for our ride. They were simple tasks, yet they were packed full of opportunities to slow down, pay special attention to details, and take time to bond with my horse. Jenny spoke about creating a connection to Duke and how he could sense everything that I was feeling. I couldn't fake a feeling with my horse, and our mutual trust was important, especially when it came to jumping.

On the day I was thrown, Jenny had decided to switch up our fences to barrels, something that Duke and I had never jumped before. I questioned her switch, and for the first time, I could actually taste fear. I had been afraid before, of things like the dark, a horror movie, or spooky camp stories, but this fear was different. This time, I was the one holding the reins.

Circling the field in warm-up, I looked at the barrel, then at my mom watching. My hands trembled. Jenny gave me last-minute instructions and then the command to face the barrel head on. Duke and I took off and gained speed. I sat up in my two-point stance and looked directly at the central point while squeezing my legs, Duke's signal to go. But right as we approached the barrel, Duke came to a screeching halt and sent me flying. I landed hard, my breath gone. Jenny ran, gave me a quick body scan, then yelled, "Get back up! Up, Ashley, get up! Try again. You already know what it's like to fall off, now try again to jump that barrel."

So, I did as I was instructed. I reached out to Duke and saddled up. Duke sensed my fear. I knew then that if I was going to clear this barrel, I would have to leave that fear behind me, focus on my goal, and make the jump while standing tall in my stands.

I took a deep breath, settled my body and my focus, and bent down and whispered to Duke, "We've got this." Together we had jumped many fences, and this was just another one. My eyes locked on the barrel, I stood determined in my two-point, and with strong legs and a deep exhale, we headed straight for it. I now knew fear and how to conquer it, just like Duke and I conquered that barrel.

The power of storytelling spans the lifeline of human beings. We learn from these stories, preserve our cultures, and provide wisdom in each story we share. History was written by the authors of it and is told by storytellers and witnesses.

We all have a story to tell. It is one of the many common threads we all share—as humans, as women. In these chapters, I share personal stories throughout my lifetime and the many journeys I've traveled. I've learned lessons from mentors and role models, life experiences and transitions. Through them, I've learned how to get back up and dust myself off. Through them, I've become the woman I am today. My story is like no other, yet it is eerily similar to those of every woman. It is the female experience.

Alongside my memories and moments are eighteen women and their stories of the female experiences that shape and connect us. To understand the female experience, we need to create the space to openly share our bravest, most vulnerable, and powerful stories. Like artist and author Morgan Harper Nichols says, "Tell the story of the mountain you climbed. Your words could become a page in someone else's survival guide."

Our stories share the wisdom of what it means to grow up female and how our self-worth supported us through the darkest of the dark and the brightest of the bright. My hope is that you will see and identify within your own life experiences the underlying current and pattern that got you through to the other side.

The power of a book's cover is that at first glance, it only reveals merely a glimpse of what you will find in the interior, much like a first impression of someone. For the whole story, you must open the book, read the chapters, and like with the overlapping petals of a peony, explore the layers that the main character has experienced: the journey of great moments, heartaches, victories, and defeats. It is only then that you might have a better understanding of who that person is at their core.

Introduction

"Ashley, it doesn't matter if you complete the race. You have already proven to everyone, including yourself, that you cannot only run it, but you can also put all of this together. You don't have to run."

Grit is a mixture of passion, perseverance, and endurance. In many situations, stories, and races, I tested my grit and found myself on the other side of the finish line. I knew failure and what it felt like to quit. I'd given up on completing a task or a challenge that spoke to my ego and proved to be stronger than my willpower. I've also tasted the sweet sweat of victory and accomplishment. The duality of life is just that: triumphs and trials, all of which are learning opportunities for me. And that Friday morning I was in a straight-up conflict over which one I would choose to put my energy into. Determination or stubbornness are so close yet very different.

As much as I loved, and often relied on, my husband Darryl's encouraging words, we both knew I was running that race despite my pulled hamstrings. I called up my running extraordinaire friend

Jenn for help. Her field of genius: running. Her line of work: physiotherapy. I heard the concern in her voice, as it matched the concern in Darryl's. They often work together in supportive roles. She told me the stretches to do, how to "mend the injury," and then in her stern words, her advice. I took it all in, including her words of wisdom, and ended the call by saying, "Don't worry, I've got this!"

I had been running for months. I'd clocked in an amazing number of hours running. I loved it. It was my form of meditation. To me, it was the best practice to fuel my mind with new ideas for work. Plus, it's quality "me time." Since the previous spring season, I had been dedicated to providing the best run and yoga series for the women of my community.

My job, along with my own passion, brought these women not only the love of the sport but also the community, connections, and friendships that come with it. I created events, socials, and activities—I loved anything that brought women together. My friend Magda once called me "a true ambassador and warrior for women."

My zone of genius is bringing women together. I've created the Kula that I spent my whole life looking for. *Kula* is a Sanskrit word that denotes a community of influential, widespread, legendary women coming together to celebrate inclusivity and a sense of belonging. I adore the world I've created. I am in every sense of the branding of Girl Time Inc. a trailblazer, forging the way with the grand visions of creating a community.

Together, the women of the Kula and I ran three times a week. I added in cross-training and yoga practice in between runs, and I fell in love with our quality time. We were a crew. Leading up to race day, I trusted that my lungs were strong, my body could and would handle the distance, and my confidence in my ability to complete my first 21 km run was set in stone. I had a goal of completing the race in two hours and ten minutes—a goal that reflected the year, the distance, and the time. Details like this mattered to me. And for this race, it was also an event that my company, Girl Time Inc., was brave enough and strong enough to pull off during the dark period of COVID-19. I was not only a runner but also the event organizer and the company backing, sponsoring, promoting, and putting on the race. To my Kula of women running beside me, I was their leader.

At our previous Thursday's group run, a run that was supposed to be "go at your own pace, nice and easy," my excitement, energy rush, and overwhelm of the list of "get to dos" had me running too hard and too fast without a conscious awareness in my strides out of the gate. The first 50 meters out, I pulled both hamstrings. I knew the damage was done. I felt it.

Aware of my injury and that the race had to carry on, I spent all of Friday resting, stretching, and abiding by my doctor's and physio's orders. Watching the clock tick closer to Saturday morning was just as painful as my pulled hamstrings. Sure enough, Saturday morning arrived, and so did my mom to help care for my kids and our puppy.

To Darryl and Jenn (and myself), I said I would start and only run what my body could handle. In a cheeky kind of way, I told them, "Guys, running is twenty percent physical and eighty percent mental." They called me stubborn, and I corrected them with a smile and a wink: "No, I'm determined! I love challenges, and this is one of them."

Wearing numerous hats comes naturally to me, and this event required me to use all my degrees and education. I am a teacher, coach, personal trainer, interior designer, event planner, facilitator, and liaison to fabulous fun. This series, like all the other events, socials, and activities I've planned, was my responsibility. The difference in this one, however, was that I was also the runner, and running the 21 km was supposed to be the easy part.

I had worked for months to pull off this race event. It was October 2021 and COVID was still very much alive. I'd opened the doors to Girl Time Inc. on June 1, 2020, right in the heat of the global pandemic. But there I was, setting up a business that sparked joy, support, and connection for women and women in business in my area. I found a way to create connection through running, hiking, and collaborating with female-led businesses to create online masterminds, workshops, book clubs, and even dinner dates. I tried any and every idea that would bring women together.

Like with this race, I had to at least try. The women who had just completed the Fall Run & Yoga series with Girl Time Inc. counted on me to bring them what I'd promised. My words mean everything to me. They're my backbone, what I stand up straight for. When I say I'm going to do something, I do it, so this race was so much more than a race—it was my warrior status in direct action.

I understood my level of pain from my hamstrings but also the pain of what we, as a collective, had and still were experiencing with the stresses and disconnection caused from the many seasons of COVID. To be human is to connect, and our connection was being blocked by the rules, regulations, and color zones built by a society and social constructions that influenced deep pain and fear in people. So, I started to put this into perspective. I asked myself, "Can I be with this pain right now? Can I fuel my body with light and ask it to carry me over the kilometers I am about to run and for the purpose I am seeking?"

I closed my eyes, re-grounded my energy, and as I breathed into these questions, I saw the bigger picture. In these moments of stillness, the lesson spoke to me: the only way is through. When we don't run into the future with our pain, we arrive with it. Moment by moment, we settle into the pain with the realization that we can "just be" with it, one moment at a time. My mantras of "just breathe" and "a body in motion, stays in motion" were on constant replay in my thoughts.

I released the pressure and sat in an honest moment of recognizing the storm (a.k.a. "the pain") I was experiencing. The storm was not about running with pulled muscles, it was about clearing the story I had carried with me since I was a child—the story that I didn't belong, that I wasn't accepted, and that I couldn't find my place. Throughout many phases in my life, I've felt the weight of insecurities and the limiting story of not being accepted for being myself, nor have I belonged to any group of women. Like a butterfly, I fluttered, always looking for it: the connection. It's the same storm that so many women are experiencing in their own way.

Whether it was the isolation of COVID or my newfound awareness, these "storms" of self-doubt and fears connected to approval, belonging, and judgment were brought to the surface. I confronted this story and said aloud, "Enough is enough." That day, the day of the race, brought me to a new place of acceptance with myself and my self-worth. *I am important. I do belong here, and I have the strength to lead others into that knowing and light.*

From this place, I asked myself for the qualities I would need to endure the run. "Is it fearlessness or softness? Is it bravery or grit? Is it courage or understanding? What is the lesson that I am seeking to move forward with more grace? Is it a combination of all the above?" In the end, regardless of the answer, the lesson always pointed back to my self-worth.

This is what these life lessons teach us. It is our return to ourselves. We fill ourselves with the light of seeing who we truly are and who we can be. It's our version of home. The connection, sense of belonging, and community support that I was seeking were found in that light and in all the actions I had put forth that got me to that race that morning. I was never without it. The story that I had been telling myself for almost forty years was the face of my fear and pain, and it was holding me back. That day, running each kilometer, I ran through the fear and the pain. My higher self and my Kula of women encouraged me to finish that race.

Jenn walked me through a proper warm-up and asked me for my clipboard. With a little nudge she said, "Go be the runner now, not the role of the director." All the ladies were arriving, ready to run either a 5 km, 10 km, or a 21 km. For some of them, this would be the first time that they had ever run a race. For others, it was a distance they were out to conquer. Regardless of the distance, thirty-five women were ready to run together and were waiting for me to give the signal to start. Switching gears, I encouraged myself to just make it to the 5 km mark. My best friend, Jen, who I'd been calling Flinty, would be there waiting. Goal number one: just run to her.

Off I went. I reached the 5 km mark, high-fived Flinty, and kept going. I headed toward the 10 km marker where Darryl and the doctor on site for the race were positioned. Reaching the marker, I smiled, mouthed the words "I love you; I've got this," and continued in the loop back to the start. At each marker I refocused and returned to my purpose and my job. My pain came in waves. "It's 80 percent mindset, 20 percent physical" was on repeat. I kept saying to myself, "I am the master of my own life experience. Let the wave go through me." I asked myself to rise above the pain and decided to release control and go with the flow.

At around the 16 km mark, my mind told me to stop. Fear was speaking louder than my hamstrings. But I didn't stop. I trusted my legs, my willpower, and most importantly, my body. Rounding the end of the race, I was now beside all the other ladies in the 5, 10 and 21 km distances. We were pointed in the direction of victory, and that energy alone was fueling me to continue. I needed to see this through for HER, for the Kula, and for myself.

At one point or another, we have experienced this feeling: the feeling of conquering something that is bigger than ourselves. It is a feeling that connects us and one that we were born having. That is the feeling of self-worth—a sense of inner confidence, plus an individual's definition of success and the ability to love ourselves and love others. It is everything we need to complete any challenge, any heartache, the dark times, and the struggle. Self-worth shows up equally in the light times, the glory, the celebrations of life achievements, goals, and triumphs. It is already inside of us. We are worthy of everything our hearts desire.

In the female experience, we can recall countless moments and memories when we were tested. We know the times of trial and defeat, and internal and external challenges of all kinds. We've experienced the sister wounds: the heartache and betrayal caused by our sisters, girlfriends, and women in our communities. We know the catcalls, and we walk to our cars with keys in our hands. We know what it is like to not believe in our capacities or capabilities. We experience limiting beliefs, impostor syndrome, self-doubt, and—wait for it—"ugly" feelings and triggers.

We have questioned our ability to love and/or our worthiness to be loved. We've been in situations where we don't feel like we belong or are accepted. We have hung our head low and have done the lonely walk of shame. We've been sexualized and mistreated; we've had our boundaries overstepped and our respect lost, simply because we are a girl. We have felt confusion, anger, and judgment triggered by hearing the words "be a good girl." We've been labeled and judged for everything that makes us an individual, and we've been cast out because of it. The female experience is real, and it has touched us all. It's part of our rite of passage.

We also know the opposite: the duality of being female. At one point or another, you felt the love and support that you can only receive from another female. There is power and truth to women supporting women. It is real. You know the magic that women have when they come together. Women's abilities to problem solve, to show up for each other, to kick ass and take names afterward. We know who our "ride or die" girlfriends are, and we call them first. They are the friends who show up with a shovel, a getaway car, and a wicked smile. They ask zero questions.

Best friends, all kinds of friendships, other girls and women who hold sacred your most cherished stories, memories, and secrets—they are the friends who created them with you. We have all reached out for the comfort and embrace from our soul sisters who hold us in a way that settles all our worries, lessens our pain, and loves us even when we are in dark places. This sisterhood love is like no other, and it is worth fighting for.

Our stories are more alike than different. There is a common pattern that we all go through when we set out to go through this journey we call life. The pattern may change in its details and in female to female, but the concrete evidence is strong. The pattern starts with self-worth.

As I turned the corner toward the last kilometer of that race, my mission was clear. I understood who I was and what I was there to do. I could clearly see the path ahead of me, and I knew I was the right girl for the job. It was time to connect and build the bridge.

I saw the families, the fellow runners, the race tent, and my son, Everett, standing with my parents. He was waving at me, encouraging me to continue going. My legs felt tired but strong. I was strides away from the finish line when Everett came running out to be beside me to the finish where my daughter, Lillian, was waiting to greet me with my medal.

My children being there and witnessing it all reaffirmed everything. They are and will forever be my most powerful WHY. The "why" I do what I do and whom I do it for. It's my heart's desire for them to grow up in a world where they know their worth, they feel a proud sense of self-belonging, and they have acceptance for all that they are: uniquely unique. All the life lessons of what it means to grow up as a female will be passed on to them in the hope that they recognize the power of their self-worth, their voice, their choices, and how much they are loved.

Race day was special. I finished in two hours and ten minutes, just as I set out to do. I felt supported by my team, my friends and family, my Kula, and my husband and kids. All the women who ran that day were victorious, and we celebrated their huge individual and group achievement. I left that event feeling confident, successful, and loved. And my biggest takeaway was the deep knowing that it is my self-worth that makes me powerful and unstoppable.

To know and share our histories and stories is to know and understand aspects of the female experience. The shared journeys and pathways we have walked, the triumphs and tragedies and how they all come together to paint a picture—those are our shared experiences. That is when you can connect the dots along our timelines and see the pattern.

To be witness to my life's connected dots and timeline is to understand why I do what I do, how I can do what I do, and the importance of what I do for you, for HER, and for us. It takes the first impression to a whole other depth of understanding the many layers of my life.

In order to do that, I must step back to the beginning of my story.

YOURstory

"Whether you think you can or you think you can't, you're right," a quote commonly attributed to Henry Ford, is a powerful one. The power is in the belief. That race would have looked completely different if I had not truly believed I could run it.

REFLECTION:

What "beliefs" do you have in yourself that get you through any and every difficult challenge? Do you have a mantra that inspires, pushes, and gets you past the edge of difficulty?

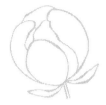

Chapter 1: Birth of a Girl

"Holy shit, Ashley . . . what have you done?" The words rolled right out of his mouth as he stared at the cast-iron hand of a wall clock piercing through my bottom lip, blood pouring down my chin. I was just three years young and in shock over what had just happened.

Our living room had had an open concept with a seating area, a dining room, and a front entrance with a large closet. It was the perfect space for small children to run, dance, play, and build up their confidence with speed drills! On the day of my accident, my mom had been out of the house (a rarity) getting her hair permed, and my dad had been left in charge of looking after the four of us: my two older sisters, my baby brother, and me. A busy job for anyone.

Typically, my dad could be found in his office, working away at building a family business from the ground up—the real traditional side of boot stampin'. The word *quit* did not exist in his world. He was a "work hard" and "play hard" kind of man and father, and whatever work–life balance he'd struck, I could always rely on him showing up for my siblings and me. But in the panicked moment with the clock, me covered in blood, he was put to the test.

Just minutes before my injury, my sister Sarah and I had decided that jumping on the couch was our next best idea for entertainment. Our eldest sister, Jessica, was playing quietly, and our baby brother, Justin, was snuggled in his rocker.

A wall clock, with two cast-iron hands and a missing glass barrier, hung above the couch where Sarah and I, laughing and jumping faster and harder, were not paying any attention to anything. As a bold, adventurous, all-in-or-all-out kind of child, I jumped higher and higher until, sure enough, I hit the clock and the long iron hand went straight through my bottom lip. Just in time, Sarah caught the clock, and together, we turned toward my dad. Holy shit indeed.

Sarah held onto the clock while my dad surveyed the scene. He called the salon, then managed to collect all of us while we waited for my mom to return home, hair still wet. A true divide-and-conquer moment. One had to stay with my baby brother and sisters, while the other took me to get stitches in my lip. This was not a typical accident, but it also wasn't my first trip to the hospital.

My dad said, "You were as calm as a cucumber. You were in control and knew you were safe with me. It wasn't until the doctor gave the order to the nurses to wrap you, to constrain you in the blanket so that he could stitch your lip without freezing, that you lost it. No one would ever hold you down."

Screaming, kicking, and causing a real fuss, I fought with marathon energy and strength. As the nurses complied and tried to hold me down, my dad snapped. He told off the doctor, swear words and all, and demanded they provide the novocaine. He knew how to calm me, how to settle my energy. Soon after, I released my fight response and stared right through the doctor and gave him permission to stitch my lip.

I wouldn't go as far to say that I was an accident-prone child, although the scar on my bottom lip (and other similar stories of injuries) might prove otherwise. I was quick to act and trusted that I could handle whatever I got myself into, as my inner sense of confidence continued to form. I walked early, talked early, and in my toddler phase, I worked hard to keep up with my two older sisters. None of this was surprising to my family. They knew who I was from day one of my life.

As the story goes, I was delivered fast and furious and came out screaming! I was seven pounds, eleven ounces, and had a set of lungs that let out a thunderous roar that reached every room on the hospital maternity floor. I certainly announced my grand entrance into the world. I was loaded with personality right from the beginning, and everyone knew it.

My parents beamed with a different kind of pride when they shared my birth story. To me, it made me feel special. Apparently, all the nurses were astonished by the power of my lungs. Even though I was tiny with little fingers, little toes, and little features including my nose, I had a presence in the room that took up the whole space. I was born with a voice; I had a story to live and then to tell.

My mother was the first to hold me. Although I was still screaming, my mom marveled over my size, my full head of jet-black hair, and my strength. She then placed me in my father's hands, a perfect fit, and in that moment, two things happened: I stopped crying, and I stole his heart. I was soothed by his voice, his strong demeanor.

My mom laughed as she told me, "I think he met his match when he met you. You held him accountable; he didn't know what hit him. You were vocal, you sought his attention, and when he would come home, you wanted to be with him, held by him. You got strength from him, but it was a different type of strength. You were his 'sweet baby doll.' He didn't think you were capable of anything bad. You were so tiny and he felt he had to protect you."

It was only when I was not busy or entertained and became bored with idle time that my demanding characteristics appeared. I'd put my feet sternly on the ground, then speak my truth in a way loud enough for them to hear. I took claim over whatever it was that I needed or wanted. I certainly had strong characteristics.

My mother openly compared me with my sisters. She didn't shy away from stating the facts to me: "You were completely opposite of your sisters: you were born screaming, they were silent; you were tiny, they were big; you had a voice and used it, they had each other. You, my third child, you changed and challenged everything! Oh, Ashley, you looked small, but you were strong. You stole the hearts of many right from the beginning."

My oldest sister, Jessica, was quiet and shy and had a temperament that ranged from slow-burn patience to quick-switch temper and mastermind. She felt the responsibility of being the older sister. She was a "mother hen," as well as a teacher and protector. Our mom often heard her say, "Don't touch that, or that, and definitely don't pull on the kitty." Jessica had to share her toys, her routine, her time, and our parents' love and attention.

Sarah, the second born, was my playmate. She loved to sing, dance, and dress up and put on a show. To me, she was the fun, outgoing one. She "spoke my language" and sparked my energy and attention! Sarah and I were active and engaged, and we explored our worlds in similar ways.

When Justin was born, the dynamics shifted. Because I admired the relationship and connection that Jessica and Sarah had with one another, I desperately wanted a little sister to call my own. After hearing the news that my parents were expecting another baby, I waited patiently, or as patiently as any toddler can, for my other half.

I made my feelings known when I learned that instead of the sister I yearned for, I had a baby brother. I took one look at him and demanded that they take him back. I didn't know it at that time that he was what I'd been looking for. He was that little sibling that I could love, loved me in return, and wanted to play! As he grew, he continued to keep up with my energy. Justin was so much more than just my little brother—he was someone I could care for, look after, protect and find a playmate in—he was exactly what I had hoped for.

As a young girl listening to my parents talk about my birth story, who I was as a baby, and the relationships I had with my siblings (my first relationships), I felt proud of all my strengths and characteristics. The list of descriptive words my mother used to describe me—*demanding, fiery, expressive, persistent, inquisitive, determined*—were not words from fairy-tale books or movies about princesses.

In hearing the stories about me as a child, I could tell that social constraints and all the expectations of how I should behave or what I "should" do as a girl had no bearing on me yet. I was confident in who I was, what I wanted, how I would make it happen, and about what success looked like once I achieved my goal. I didn't know how to put on the breaks or hide myself. I loved my uniqueness and didn't question it. It all made perfect sense to me.

My ideas of belonging and understanding who I am as a person would come from my early experiences with my family, in recognizing who my parents were and are, and through my socialization with my siblings. These are infinite lessons that children, baby girls, learn right from the beginning and answer everything later.

According to my mom, I was an observant child. I watched and was highly stimulated by my sisters' play. They would sing and dance around and entertain me while I clapped and giggled and was happy and content. But that changed when I wanted something and was no longer entertained. Mom said, "Halfway was never good enough for you—you had to have it all and that is when you were demanding."

A fight between sisters is like wild cats in the jungle: screaming, demanding, stomping, yelling, crying. Even though I was younger, I never bowed my head; I rose to the battle. I gave it just as I received it, and in many instances, I became bigger, stronger, and laid it all out for them; I was fierce. I demanded to be heard just as much as they did. My parents had no choice but to intervene. Our mom usually handled the screaming matches, but one time in particular, our dad stepped in. He divided us with his voice of authority: "Ashley, that is enough! You are a lion, and she is a sheep. You are too strong. Now go! Off you go." This is my first recollection of the lesson on playing small. Lions are shot in spaces that protect sheep.

Soon after, commands, expectations, and corrections about how to behave as a little girl began appearing. Our mom, after getting us ready for the day with perfect outfits, perfect shoes, and perfect hair, would give directional cues: "Stand up straight, shoulders down. Get that out of your mouth. Don't touch your sister. Stop arguing with each other. Smile. Ashley, children are a direct reflection of their parents. Now, do your best to behave. Think before you do. Think before you say, and please, remember who your family is."

As a young girl, I modeled what I was seeing and experiencing from my own world, and that fueled my dreams for my own future. My biggest "little girl" dream was motherhood. Oh how I wanted to be a mom. I absolutely loved playing with dolls and truly felt connected to the experience of pretending to be a mom. I took my "babies" everywhere, and if they needed to be changed, I would stop, drop what I was doing, and take care of that. If they were hungry, I would pull up my shirt and pretend to breastfeed.

With my Barbies, I acted out different lifestyles, imaginary situations, and conversations, again modeling what I was seeing, hearing, and witnessing in my world. One of my favorite storylines included Barbie "having it all": the house, the car, the clothes, the shoes, the accessories. She was rich, had a ton of friends, and was dating the most handsome man. Jobwise, she was a businesswoman. Barbie always had a party to go to and always in a new dress. Her handsome man was a professional too, either a businessman, lawyer, or doctor depending on the day of play. He was distinguished, sophisticated, and well liked, and was a doting partner. Barbie always married the man and always had children, but her babies just slept so they didn't interrupt her lifestyle or nightlife.

I loved play like this. My imagination was strong, and I could truly lean into the scenario that I had created for either my Barbies or my dolls. By this time, though, unless I had a playdate with a school friend or my cousin Meghan, I was playing dolls and Barbies by myself. My sisters had no interest in playing with me, and if we did attempt to play, we did not connect to each other's storyline or imagination.

I remember one time in particular, while playing Barbies solo, I was pretending that Barbie went to the hair salon. Out of all the Barbies that my sister Jessica and I had combined, I selected Jessica's Barbie to go to the salon and cut her Barbie's hair right off, right down to the doll's scalp.

Intentionally, Barbie looked like the late Irish singer–songwriter Sinead O'Connor. At that time, my mom had been inspired by Sinead's iconic hairstyle: the shaved head on a female was an act of sovereignty to herself and to the public; it was a rebellion. For whatever reasons my mom had, she shaved her head and wore it proudly. Naturally, so did my Barbie. I LOVED it!

But when Jessica found her Barbie with this new hairstyle, she lost her mind. She was beyond furious with me. She had already, on several accounts, made it very known that she hated cleaning up after me and playing and caring for me, and now I had just destroyed her Barbie. To her, this was intentional Barbie butchery, a true act of malice. To me, it was Barbie being rebellious, fashionable, and Sinead O'Connor.

We never played Barbies together again. I was given strict rules not to touch Jessica's Barbies or any of her belongings, guidelines that I somewhat respected but occasionally ignored when a friend or Meghan came over. I wasn't allowed to touch her Barbies, but there was never any mention of them not being allowed in group play.

I knew I was growing up when my interests started to change along with the storyline for my Barbies. As I changed and matured, so did Barbie's life. Barbie's life began to include conflicts and fights between Barbie friends. Barbie play no longer focused on her getting married; instead, it was focused on proms, boyfriends, and shopping. Barbie was "younger" and childless.

Together with my friends, our play had shifted focus. We explored the role of "businesswomen" while playing in my dad's office. I would sit at his desk—the boss's desk—and make pretend calls, do pretend paperwork, and sometimes, even pretend to hire or fire people. We knew how to work the photocopier and make coffee, so we took our dedication to our imagination a step further and drank the coffee too. I had a team of workers who I would assign "jobs" to while pretending to guide them through the procedures and tasks assigned.

I was the boss. In that imaginary world, I could be a lioness. My friends loved it too. We felt powerful. We were in charge of our own world and were unstoppable in the businesses that we created. My dad's store, a flooring, drapery, and decor store, had all the materials imaginable to create "mood boards," so I had a new form of play that ignited my creative side: I would pretend I was an interior designer, a famous one!

This new space was ours to explore, create, and take our imaginations anywhere in the world. No one was supervising us, which gave us the opportunity to be silly, be bold, be anything we wanted to be. And at the end of our playdates, I would pack up, turn off the lights, and tell my pretend secretary, "I'll handle it all in the morning. I'm going home to my family."

YOURstory

Birth charts, human design, our thumbprints: they all show how uniquely different we are. Our experiences and descriptive words describing our personalities and characteristics may be similar, but we are not created from the same cookie cutter. Your self-image is an important one to discover.

REFLECTION:

What words do you use to describe who you were as a child and who you are now? What similarities and differences do these words have to each other?

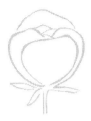

Chapter 2:
The Search for Identity

Around the age of nine, my hair was long, thick, and beautiful. I loved wearing sparkly makeup, blue eyeshadow, and dresses. Any event was a reason to dress up. Female curves and breasts hadn't started to develop on me yet, but the idea of developing boobs, and big boobs at that, to fill in the fancy dresses was ideal. At Devon's birthday party, my childhood best friend, I stuffed a pair of water balloons in my swimsuit and proudly walked around as if they were real breasts. All the other girls giggled as I strutted around, feeling beautiful and very grown up.

The fall I was going into fourth grade, my mom signed me up to be a child hair model. I had modeling experience, as Mom had signed my siblings and me up for modeling before when she was working for a children's clothing store downtown. We dressed the part, smiled, and did the walk. This time around, though, the hair salon had brought in a professional hair stylist from the city to show all the small-town stylists new trends.

The stylist asked me if I knew the music group Wilson Phillips. Instantly, I relaxed, and I started singing their songs. They were one of my favorite musical groups—strong female singers whose lyrics were inspiring and positive and represented dreams that I wanted to someday obtain. Before the stylist began the haircut, he informed me that he was going to model it after the lead singer. He stepped away, spoke with my mom, then in one swift motion, he tied my long hair up in a high ponytail and cut it all off.

I went from having hair touching my butt to a mushroom cut. GONE. It was all gone. I couldn't grasp what he had just taken from me. Red-hot panic flashed through my body, my brain quickly asked a million questions, and all I wanted to do was hide. Instead, I hung my head, covered my face, and cried.

Everyone was in shock. When we arrived at home, my dad didn't even recognize me. "Kath, who's that kid?" he asked my mom. At school, all my friends, classmates, and teachers had a comment, and none of them were good. Suddenly I was being teased at school. I was told I looked like a boy, that I was ugly. At recess, the name calling, shame, and embarrassment over my new tomboy haircut caused a shift in my behavior and play.

Bully mentality showed up many times after that haircut. One boy in particular targeted me and made me the butt of every joke he made. At swimming lessons, he held me under the water. His sick game created my new fear of drowning. During recess, he cornered me between the fence lines, pointed, laughed, and made fun of my haircut and now another new "imperfection," my nose. I was so beyond done. I had spoken up, had told my teachers and my parents and had asked for help, yet nothing stopped him. Panic and anger felt the same to me. But this time, this day at the fence, instead of crying and trying to hide, I stood up and kicked him square in the "round tables." It was my first fight and I felt a new kind of confidence. The boy ran after me, but now I was the one smiling for I knew I could outrun and outsmart him, duck away and blow past him. I was faster, smaller, and feistier. I had my own back and that was my power.

Shortly after this notorious haircut, my first "boyfriend," the boy who gave me butterflies in my stomach, broke up with me. He didn't like my new style. It was my first heartbreak, and I walked home in tears. I now knew hatred. I had hatred for my ugly haircut, the boy who bullied me, and now, my broken heart.

The thing about change is that it is constant, a hard concept to grasp for a young girl. But once I was aware of the consistency of change, I saw it everywhere. My sister Jessica entered high school and Sarah grade eight, and I was right behind their every move. I was the witness. I watched my little brother play with the older boys and take on new experiences that he was not ready for. The word *party* was introduced and so was drinking and experimenting with drugs. Plus, a ton of new people, new friends, coming through our house doors.

My dad was always working at this time, and although my mom was there, she wasn't truly present. Her mother's health was deteriorating, which meant my mom was experiencing a whole other world of impermanence, and one that I had zero experience in, death. My grandmother Marjorie, a lady who I am proudly named after, had been diagnosed early in life with Multiple Sclerosis, an autoimmune disease that attacked her central system and caused her to lose the strength in her once-strong legs. My entire lifetime she had been in and out of the hospital and had used a wheelchair.

I never liked our trips to the hospital. I recall the long hallways, the sterile smell, and how most of the patients sat staring at their TVs or out the window. It felt lonely and distant there—a place that as a small child, I knew I never wanted to be.

With the Christmas holiday season upon us, my siblings and I were at our neighbor's house celebrating. Music was loud, and the adults were drinking, dancing, and carrying on. We, too, were dancing and laughing to the great tunes of the '70s and their funny lyrics. Everything was high energy and bright lights, until it wasn't. One phone call shut everything down.

Jackie, our neighbor, told us it was time to go home and be with our mom, that she needed us and had news. Jackie was one of the most magical people I knew, always full of wild energy, and this phone call had made her instantly sober and serious. I had been a part of Jackie's family as their babysitter for a couple of years and was aware of her energy shifts. I could tell by the tone of her voice that something bad had happened.

We trekked through the snow toward home. There was only one light on, and even it was dimmed. Our home felt off; something was missing and cold. We were greeted by my dad, and he whispered that our grandmother had passed away and our mother was devastated. We were not allowed to go into their bedroom; rather, we needed to get our rest. The next day would be long and tiring for everyone.

My mom wore a long black taffeta skirt and shirt outfit with white pearls to the funeral, and although the light had gone out of her eyes, she still looked beautiful and serene. She held herself with poise, remained well mannered, and was somehow taller than usual. My siblings and I dressed, black shoes and coordinated, and on the drive to the church, no one spoke. I just witnessed the slight moves, teardrops, and the echoing silence of grief, a foreign concept, settling in. The topic of death had never been discussed in our house before. I watched as my parents greeted the family, my grandpa, and their close friends. I could tell by my mom's facial expressions, mannerisms, and words that she was making everyone comfortable while holding in her own emotions. It was yet another example of constraint and a new meaning to the word *hold*.

My mom did not crack; she held it together and looked at us to follow. At many funerals, people mourn the loss of their loved one and weep together in community. This was not the case for us. My siblings and I were to be stoic, calm, quiet, and put together. I held my breath for what seemed like the entire day that day. Inside, all I wanted to do was cradle my mom. Instead, I followed in line.

As I continued to grow older, female role models were everywhere. Jackie, my teachers, my riding and dance instructors, my aunts, my grandmother, and my mom—I was always watching them and taking mental notes. I saw that my mother wore all the hats. She was in charge of running our house and home and caring for four children—four different stages, ages, personalities, and characteristics—a 24/7 job that didn't come with a paycheck but required every ounce of her, even as she was grieving the loss of her own mother and dealing with family drama that came with her burial.

Change brought dark times to my home's doorstep, and I noticed. The shadow touched everything. The socioeconomic struggles that were happening during the '80s and '90s impacted small businesses, which included my father's. He was building a business, bottom to his version of top, something that took a ton of his energy, focus, and time. I watched him from the window of our front living room. His office was only steps away—our neighboring property. At his desk, he had laser focus: he had goals to achieve plus the weight of having four children and all our needs. These were big concepts that I understood very little about. All I knew from my childlike observations was that Dad was stressed and Mom was hanging on.

Patience, stillness, and when to pause; readiness, embrace, and when to go—all these life lessons were teaching me oppositional balance. With light there is dark, with right there is wrong, with up there is down, with inhale there is exhale, with sunshine there is rain . . . where there is life, there is death. This is life's balance, and it is always in a constant state of motion. The list of opposites continues, and so do their powerful counterpoints. They bring the scales to perfect alignment, measuring equally the weight of each other. That is the duality of this world.

At a time when I was just starting to figure out who I was becoming, what I liked and disliked, our roles within a family unit, friendships, and their value, I began clearly understanding that nothing ever stayed the same and that everything has an opposite. I witnessed the hold that grief had on my mom, the stressors of being a businessman on my father, and the changes that come with adolescence and maturity with my two older sisters. Somewhere in that, I understood "dark times."

But where there is dark, there is light. I remember the day I heard the music before I saw the car: a forest-green Mustang GT convertible with a tan roof in all its glory, and my parents in theirs. The sun was shining, the car—this magnificent piece of metal—was gleaming, and the smiles on my parents' faces were beaming for all to see. They had made the choice to act in their dark times and be the spark that would bring light. It was a lighthouse moment for anyone experiencing the storm.

This car represented their hard work within the home and in the family business. It sparked joy after experiencing great loss. My parents showed us strength in their solidarity and that the only way to the other side is by going through. That day, that memory, planted a seed in my heart and a fire in my soul. It was a lesson, a goal, and a promise to myself that I, too, would one day know that glory, and until then, I would work for it. This was my first taste of defining success to myself. Mustang Sally, as we called it, became so much more to me than a car. It was a symbol of hope, a rush of speed, the hard work of determination. It ignited the desire to live in the fast lane and a goal for a life full of inspiration. Its purpose was to spark joy, laughter, and fun.

And it did just that. On a trip in the Mustang to my cousin's house one weekend, my dad told me that we were on a joyride. The top was down, my hair was blowing in every direction, and our music was loud. I looked at my dad and saw rejuvenation. I could see him breathing differently, as though he was as light as a feather and in his element of play. Dad gave me the look: "Hold on!" then shifted gears and put the pedal to the floor. Eleven cars and trucks—we passed them all, and I experienced a new form of glory, freedom, and success. This car would be in my future. I was maturing at a rapid rate, and these were the big lessons that I was taking with me.

As my dad drove past the eleven cars, I realized that I, too, was passing into my eleventh birthday and my needs and wants, as well as my heart's desires, were changing just as fast. I was discovering who I was becoming, and my sense of self was being challenged by what I thought before and what I would think next. Would anything stay the same? Could I slow down time or take a moment to process what was happening before it all happened to me?

HERstory

KRISTEN

"My mother passed away from cancer two days before her forty-first birthday. I was six years old. One day she was struggling to get out of bed. What felt like the next day, she was a stone box of ashes. I never had the opportunity to say goodbye to her; I didn't understand death at that age. No one was there to teach me how to grieve for my mother."

Kristen's first love was her mother, and this love started in her mother's womb, a space where she felt cared for, nurtured, safe, and warm. When she was born, she knew love before she knew any other emotion. Before the world and people who surrounded her told her, showed her, taught her, and treated her any differently, she knew love.

Children have the most innocent sense of love from and fear of other people. It is the purest sense of self that directs them to the people they can trust and take safety in and love in return.

Kristen knew this love. She counted on it. To her, her mother was her everything. Her early childhood source of love, comfort, and nurturing came solely and directly from her mother. She also knew the complete opposite: disconnection and fear from an emotionally immature and physically abusive father. A young child, very new to the world, still knew the difference between love and fear.

A few weeks after Kristen turned six, her safety net—her sense of love, comfort, nurturing, and security—was gone when her mother passed away from cancer. One day she was there and the next, she wasn't. Suddenly Kristen's world completely changed, and not for the better.

Kristen had her sister, aunt, uncle, and father. Stunned and silent, they felt as if everything had paused as they stared blankly at each other and tried to process what had happened and how the world would continue without Kristen's mom. Kristen sat at the front of the funeral home and watched as people approached the platform and shared stories about her mother, stories that did not connect with Kristen for she did not know this other side of her mom. These people could have been talking about a stranger for all she knew. The reference to an angel was on repeat: "She's in Heaven now." "She's an angel now." "She will watch over you from Heaven—a perfect angel."

Grief, the emotional suffering left when someone is taken from you, is hard enough for an adult or someone who has experience with it and an "understanding" of life. For a child, grief is very difficult to grasp, understand, and feel. It is nearly impossible to conceptualize that the person who was with you one day and not the next is now in a place that people call "Heaven"—a place no one can see, feel, touch, or that holds any sense of tangibility. To Kristen, time became obsolete—it no longer existed with the one person that made her feel safe and loved. And sadly, time had passed before Kristen could even gain the insight to hold on to with gratitude every passing second she'd had with her mother while she was alive. And due to the state of her mother's sickness and the decisions made by the adults surrounding Kristen and her sister, they never had their chance to say goodbye. Young Kristen only knew that seconds had passed, then her mother was gone.

In shock and grief, Kristen and her sister were placed in the care of their father, a man who, unfortunately, was absent when it came to nurturing them as a father who cared. Grief itself can cause erratic behavior in people, and the difference in Kristen's story is that her father already had erratic behavior while her mother was alive. In her passing, the erratic behavior increased.

Kristen knew of his temper, his aggressive outlashes, and his belligerence because of her previous experiences with him. She had been fearful of him even when her mother was still earthbound. Kristen recalled times in her childhood when she would cry, and her father's response focused only on his need to stop the sound. He often placed his hands around her throat in desperation to get her to quiet. Due to her fear, both her body and brain retained the memory of being choked, and she lost her ability to cry, to release her sadness. Kristen became mute to expressing her emotions to her father.

Kristen, a little girl processing the death of her mother, was left confused. She was surrounded by the noise of others and held the concept her mother as a perfect, flawless angel. Kristen was alone— no one got down to her level, took her by the hand, and walked her through the biggest transition of her life. All she knew was that she didn't want to be in a world where her mother wasn't. Even though she was incredibly young, Kristen questioned her existence in this world. For a little girl who hadn't grasped the impermanence of death, she understood its darkness and desired it.

"I didn't understand death. I just thought that she left us. I looked for her everywhere I went: in the grocery store, walking down the street, in crowds of people. Maybe, just maybe, it was all a joke and I would find her. Dark thoughts crept in my mind. I no longer wanted to be here—I only wanted to be with her. In hearing the words 'death,' 'died,' and 'die' without understanding them, I expressed that I too wanted to die. In pain, crying alone to my mother's urn, I just wanted to be with her. I never felt safe with my father."

After the funeral, when everyone left to go home and return to the world that never stopped, darkness slowly crept in and took over the household. No one was there to care for Kristen or her sister. It did not take long for her father to remove himself from household and parental duties. No one tucked her in at night, read her bedtime stories, or showed any form of nurture to her.

Her older sister, while experiencing her own grief and life adjustments of a young girl, fell into herself. Kristen, being a witness to it all, felt like her sister opted out of the world and their relationship. She became separate and was in her own bubble. They learned how to be alone, together. And in time, they figured out how to coexist and take on daily life. They handed each other ingredients to make meals, they tidied the house, and they slowly learned to care for each other.

But to Kristen, her mother was the only one she was seeking out. That void could not be filled by anything or anyone. She also came to understand that she needed to look for safety and security outside of the home, and her school became one of those places. She would wake up, get herself ready for the day, and make her way to the playground where she would be welcomed in. The school served as her safety net, a warm place to rely on as well as a place of structure and a practice ground for her development. It introduced her to socialization and brought her adult figures and role models.

School also had a regimented system. It was full of schedules, daily tasks, and work to be done, but it also served as a reminder that she was indeed raising herself. A simple thing such as her agenda—sent home with her homework, reading buddy tasks, and the requirement of a parent's signature—was a trigger for her. Her father was not home to sign it, or he would forget. She assumed blame for his absence, which left Kristen with a lecture from the teacher the next day. Something so simple happened over and over.

Kristen soon learned to do as she was told, to follow the rules and not upset her teacher. She began signing her own reading logs after reading aloud to her pet bunny (because there was no one else to read to). She studied, did her homework, and proved to be incredibly bright. Through these actions, Kristen gained early habits of people pleasing, all to ensure that adult figures would stay in her world.

The school system was full of opportunities to be around other people, friends, teachers, peers, and most importantly, female role models. Kristen looked for other girls, women, and female leaders to be her guides throughout her development. Her energy was naturally drawn and attracted to strong, nurturing, professional women in roles of leadership. They were the ones who took notice of her and modeled self-love and worthiness.

"There were dozens of girls and women who had a positive impact on me during my childhood and adolescence. I had babysitters who showed me how to paint nails, a friend who gave me my first bra, and a neighbor who taught me how to shave my legs and do a high ponytail. I had friends' mothers cook dinners when I visited, a teacher who cared for me like I was her own daughter, and a music instructor who paid for flute repairs. Most importantly, I had a loving sister who, still to this day, continues to inspire me with her strength, patience, and unwavering kindness."

What we seek, we find. Kristen found strong female role models and relationships everywhere she went. These women all demonstrated the strength that women hold within themselves and although none of them could or would replace the sacred space of her mother, they showed her love. Love, more powerful than fear, became Kristen's North Star as she navigated the next ages and phases of her life. Her greatest journey would be to the center of loving herself and seeing just how worthy she is of that love.

MORGAN

"I lived for mixtapes, dance parties, playing Barbies and laughing until our tummies hurt. Quality time with my family, my cousins, and my best friend is what I lived for. My childhood was full of fun-loving memories. How lucky were we? We had each other and nothing else mattered in the world."

The veil of knowledge is real for little girls. One day they are playing with dolls, Barbies, and children's toys, and the next, they question if they are still allowed to. It is an internal question, yet it is placed within the social contract on what is and is not accepted at certain ages of development. "Am I too old to play?" This is when the veil of knowledge drops and you understand that yes, you are indeed growing up and then acknowledge that change is happening within you.

The development of self—who you are, what you like, what you dislike, what brings you joy, what shuts you down—is the phase of figuring out where you belong in the world. It is also when you question whether you'll be accepted and liked for who you are.

Morgan was a shy, quiet girl at school. She recalls kids, so-called friends, making fun of her and calling her "beaver" because of her teeth. In front of them, her solution was to brush it off, walk away from it, and ignore the name calling. At home, though, she would break down and cry to her mom. Her mother's response was to repeat the saying, "sticks and stones may break my bones, but words will never hurt me." Unfortunately, words have power and they do hurt.

Morgan blossomed to her true self when she was home with her family. There, she felt the most comfortable and confident. Home was a place that she could and would be her true self. She was a little girl who loved to play Barbies and dolls, using her imagination to create any world that she wanted to be in. To her, playing Barbies allowed her to open up to what she was witnessing in life and her dreams; it allowed her to live through the fictional characters she created.

Although she lived two hours away from her first cousin, her best friend, Morgan counted the days in between the holidays when they would get an opportunity to spend quality time together, playing, laughing, dancing, and just being silly. She lived for family time. This time together filled her heart with joy.

Together, they were little girls off on adventures and living the dream life—a Barbie life full of dresses, shoes, the house, and the car. They spent hours upon hours in the sacred Barbie nook, pretending that the dolls were businesswomen, mothers, fashion designers. They also created a secret language and sent letters through the mail written in this code. Receiving a letter from one another was better than anything. They shared their dreams, their hopes, and their wishes, laughed at each other's jokes, and even coached each other through fights with their parents, first crushes, kisses, and heartaches. They spoke about when they would grow up: what it would be like and how they would find the man of their dreams, get married, have children, and drive convertibles. Never once did Morgan play in a shy, quiet, or reserved way. When in the same space, Morgan and her cousin were inseparable and on top of the world.

One day while taking the dog for a walk, they came across an electric fence and a herd of cattle. All it took was for one of them to spark the idea. They were set on proving that one cannot tip over a sleeping cow. In white jean shorts, Morgan jumped over the electric fence and headed toward the target, her cousin and the German Shepherd already ahead of her running in the field.

Just as they got close to the cattle, the dog started biting at the cows' ankles and irritated the herd enough for all of them to break out in a full run. The girls, running as fast as they could back to the fence, had the dog and the herd of cattle close behind. Unfortunately, Morgan didn't quite make it over the fence because the dog took her feet out beneath her, causing her to slip in cow shit while getting shocked by the fence. Her cousin, who had cleared the fence, rolled on the ground with laughter at the sight. But Morgan wasn't angry: they found laughter in everything, even the inappropriate and awkward things and especially when the other got hurt or made a fool out of herself.

Morgan and her cousin had a true sisterhood. They trusted each other and had an inner knowing that the other one would be there through it all. As they matured, and their bodies, interests, and hobbies changed, they had each other to confide in and share their inner thoughts, worries, and what they thought they should "be."

Life at school was changing for Morgan, as she was one of the early bloomers. Her feelings of self-consciousness developed when her breasts and a round bum did. Her early development separated her from the other girls, who were tiny and petite. She was maturing faster than everyone else, and that served Morgan with both pros and cons.

"I had to wear a training bra in grade five. Boys in my class would come and snap my bra, then run away laughing. There were only two other girls in my grade who had to wear a bra, which made us different from the other girls. I didn't mind the attention, though, as it was better than being called 'beaver.' It was something that deemed me 'cool.'"

Morgan shared all her feelings with her cousin, her upsets about the name calling and the hush-hush feelings of liking the attention from the boys and being different. She never felt judgment from her cousin, only reassured that she was heard and loved.

Although they lived hours away from one another, they found each other during all the important moments. The love they had reached the distance and made every family holiday more special, simply because they shared it together. When Morgan's parents would pack up for the weekend visits with the extended family at her grandparents' home, Morgan would light up. It was her happy place, her home. Together with all her cousins, Morgan could be herself, all of herself, and everyone loved every inch. At her grandparents' place, Morgan and her cousins played for hours on their own. The adults had trust in them, trusting that they looked out for each other and took care of one another.

Laughter filled the home. They had wild imaginations and so many games. The floor became hot lava and the only way to survive was to jump, climb, and help each other from the stairway to the other side of the room and back. In her uncle's warehouse, full of carpets and obstacles to climb on and hide in, a simple game of hide-and-go-seek quickly turned into brilliant fun for everyone to discover new hiding places. And when they were not playing in the carpets, they were pretending to be top businesswomen, sitting at the boardroom desks and making phone calls, big-business style. Playing board games, skinny-dipping in the pool, swimming in the grandparents' pond, biking at the beach, going on summer camping adventures, hiking trails, and participating in endless car games, Morgan enjoyed it all with her family.

Morgan had a special bond with her grandmother. Her grandma saw her in a different light, and time together was sacred. They spent weekends, holidays, and summer vacations together. They would go shopping; play the piano; attend church choir practice, plays, and performances; and cook and dance around the kitchen. Her grandma took her everywhere and introduced her to everyone. She made Morgan feel like the most important person in the world. She loved Morgan like no other.

To Morgan, home with her family and extended family was the best place to be and the place where she belonged. With them, she was not quiet, shy, and reserved. With them, she was exactly who she wanted to be and become. She was growing up in a nurturing and accepting home full of happy times where people wanted to be together. Here, she didn't question whether she could be ten and still play with Barbies. There was no judgment or fear of it. She was accepted; she belonged. To a little girl who was not feeling seen at school, her sense of home was found within herself and with the people who valued her. This was Morgan's place to shine—and she did!

YOURstory

A role model is someone who inspires others. They have the power of influence and leave a lasting imprint on someone else's life. Parents, teachers, family members, and friends can all be role models in a child's life and help shape their identity. Children at any age and phase look up to a variety of different role models to guide, teach, and help them learn how to engage in relationships, community, and society.

REFLECTION:

Who were your role models and what lessons did you learn from them? How did their influence impact your identity?

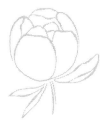

Chapter 3:
It's a Girl Thing

I loved watching old, classic movies. The older, the better. My icons were Audrey Hepburn and Vivien Leigh, and I adored all their movies, but specifically *Breakfast at Tiffany's* and *Gone with the Wind*. When my other friends were watching the popular movies of the '80s, I was back in history with these powerful women. I felt a strange connection to HER, the leading lady of that time period. I loved the culture, the building structures, and the obvious: the dresses, hats, and parties. Mainly though, I admired how the heroine demanded more of society and her roles as a woman in it. Scarlett O'Hara, for example, was bold, extremely forward, a boss lady, and very vocal; she dared to lead and was fierce and fearless. She was everything that I wanted to be. I watched how she handled herself and did not apologize for who she was, regardless of how others felt about her. She was my hero. And if I wasn't watching powerful women in film, I was watching powerful women on TV: Buffy (the Vampire Slayer), Sailor Moon, Xena (the Warrior Princess), Oprah—any and all leading ladies who were bold, brave, vocal, and determined to be heard, seen, and valued.

Sadly, regardless of the strength I found in these leading ladies, I was also watching conflicting messages about sexualization—how these and so many women on screen were dressed, how they used their femininity as a tool of seduction, and how the men treated them as a result. During this time, I was maturing, and my body was changing. I'd started to develop breasts, curves, and womanly features, and I had a curiosity that matched. And when these features started to "blossom," so did the attention from the opposite sex, attention that came with no guidance, open communication, or mentorship from any of the women in my life. It was quite the opposite, in fact. It came with competition, comparisons, shame, lack of communication, and division. I was considered "sexy," a word that even to this day makes me cringe. I still recall the day, while playing floor hockey in my dad's warehouse with my brother and his buddies, that my grandmother made a comment, one that I only fully understood later in life: "Be careful, Ashley, you have bedroom eyes and those can be used as a weapon."

I had far too many mixed messages to grasp on to for me to have a healthy self-image. I struggled to understand what a girl "should" be and who I was. The social demand to be a "good girl" meant so many conflicting things. I should be smart but not too smart that I keep down any male counterpart. I should be well read but not vocal with my thoughts and feelings, or heavens, make any demands. I should be athletic but not faster than the boys or aggressive on the soccer field. I often felt as if I were living in the same age and era of Scarlett, and I, too, wanted to not give a damn.

The summer after finishing grade six, my friend Linda and I spent a couple weeks at overnight co-ed summer camp. One of the boys there, Steve, had a huge crush on me. The problem was that Linda and another girl had a huge crush on him. It was a love triangle with a twist. I didn't like Steve, however, as he wasn't my "type." But the more attention Steve gave me, the more distance and girl drama it caused.

The day that it poured rain, right through from the night to the end of the next day, our camp turned into a huge mud pit. It was perfect conditions for a full-out mud fight for the campers and counselors, and Linda and I were right in the middle of it and loving every second. Then Steve made his move. He tackled me to the ground and professed his love. I started laughing awkwardly, not knowing how to respond. Linda thought she knew what to do: she threw a huge mud ball right at my face. I choked on the mud, and then she was the one laughing.

The girls and women in my life weren't always supportive of me. In fact, it felt like overnight I woke up to a different side of them, especially when it came to competition and comparison. And a new word entered my understanding: *threat*. I was on a different territory and had become a target.

At the beginning of grade seven, I found out quickly just how powerful feelings of *threat* would prove to be for some. A regular trip to the bathroom during class time one day turned into my being cornered by two of the grade eight girls. One of them, the ringleader and shorter of the two, demanded that I give her my shirt. She said the guy she liked noticed it and thought it would look better on her. The second girl, standing on my other side, towered over me. It was a strategic placement, a premeditated position of power and an intimidation tactic, one that I recognized, as I had two older sisters. I knew this drill. What they did not expect was that I would flatly refuse them and fire back with a "hell no!" I did not bow my head or give in to their demands. I knew that if I did not stand up to them on that day, they would keep this power position for the rest of the school year. And that was something, like my shirt, I was not about to give them.

When I got my first period, I was standing in line for gym class. I had no idea what to do, who to tell or talk to, or how I was going to survive the day. Conversations about maturity and puberty had not been a topic I'd ever discussed with my mother or older sisters. So I stuffed a shit ton of toilet paper in my underwear and prayed that I would make it through the day.

All I could think about was calling my cousin. She was the only person I ever spoke to about what was happening to me with puberty, girl drama, boy drama, and everything in between. She always had answers and would know what to do. She had already experienced her first period during the summer, and luckily, my aunt had been right there to support and celebrate her coming of age.

When I got home that day, I was full of embarrassment and ran crying to my sisters and mom. Their response was to tell me to handle it. So I called my cousin, and as expected, she walked me through maxi pads and advised me not to use tampons. That would come later.

Life moved on. Soon it was my grade eight graduation, and the night was magical for so many reasons, yet filled with a lack of communication for so many others. My graduation dress was halter-style; it was floor-length bright red satin with sparkly sequences around the neck and breast line, and I wore it confidently. My hair was done, and my mom had hired a professional makeup artist to come and complete my look. I was not a little girl anymore. I was responsible, getting good grades, making money as a babysitter, and now, graduating grade school. That night, I wore that red dress as my declaration that I was ready for and had arrived at the next phase of life.

Together with some of my classmates, we rented a limo. We wanted to arrive at our Hollywood theme dinner and graduation in style. But for some reason unbeknownst to me, my mom had arranged for my neighbor, the same age as my older sister Jessica, to accompany me to my graduation. Little did she know the dislike I had for him. In fact, it was more like hatred. He was manipulative, crossed far too many personal boundaries, was physically, mentally, and sexually abusive, and he'd increased the separation between my sister Jessica and me as a result. But there he was, smiling and asking for my hand to walk me to the limo.

I knew how to put on the face that said, "Everything is fine," as I had watched for many years how it was done. The social expectations and instructions I'd been receiving were that what you think, feel, and are experiencing deep inside are not for the public knowledge. That night, the way the neighbor looked at me in my form-fitted, red dress made my stomach turn and vomit come to my mouth: "You are so sexy," he then said. I swallowed the vomit and never mentioned out loud how uncomfortable I was or how I wanted to hide from his gaze. How I looked had suddenly become unsettling and gross.

It was yet another boundary crossed with no one to turn to for help. Apparently, I was the problem. I was the one who wore that dress, that eye shadow, and who smelled like vanilla perfume. The voice inside my head said loud and clear, "Lower your head. Don't make eye contact. It's all your fault. You are a girl and he's just being a boy; that's what they do. Hide your disgust, put on your fake smile, and get into the vehicle like a good girl." It was clear. The opportunity for communication was again missed.

The dinner and the gymnasium were decorated in the Old Hollywood theme, and each student was awarded an "Oscar" for a shining characteristic or a future ambition they had. Mine, in gold writing, said, "Future Movie Star." I was the one, just like Scarlett, in the bright red dress, stopping the crowd and making a grand entrance.

Then high school began. Everything you think about yourself is tested on the first day of high school. Decisions must be made: ride the bus or walk? Arrive in a car with friends or older siblings? What to wear, who to speak to, who to walk around with. Even what classes you're in. Everything gets judged. The answers to all of these align and point you to which social hierarchy you'll belong too. It's like herding sheep. Everyone is also curious, anxious, and even a little bit naive to the process. Including me.

When entering high school, I was already more experienced than a lot of other students, something that gave me both an advantage and a disadvantage. I was the little sister. I'd been part of the summer hot tub parties where I met a lot of my sisters' friends and acquaintances. I'd had my first kiss: a wet sloppy one in grade five. I saw drunk teens in grade seven. I knew of kids my age and older already engaged in sex and drugs. All this to say, I was not new to the scene. The difference now, though, was that I had entered a place, age, and phase where I could decide how I wanted to partake in these rites of passage of adolescent discoveries.

What I did not expect, however, was the attention I received from the boys in my grade and above. The boys I had gone to grade school with were different. There had been no dating, and if there had been, it was only for amateurs. High school opened a whole new level of dating that included no written rules, boundaries, or guidelines. And I had too much attention for anyone, especially because, being the new girl on the scene, it could and would cost me.

One thing I understood immediately was the difference between what boys could get away with and what girls definitely could not. On any given weekend party, if a girl "made out" with a guy, or worse, "went to third or fourth base," she was labeled a slut. Monday would come, and everybody and their mother knew about it. But the boy in that same situation was awarded with high fives in the hallway during break. He was revered as "a stud," "cool," a "prince." It was a terrible double standard, and to make matters worse, the girl who kissed the boy would get completely destroyed by other girls on that Monday. Rumor mills, name calling, back-stabbing, full-out chick fights—both physically and emotionally—became far more damaging than a group of boys calling her a slut.

Friends you had in grade school also changed. With every new boyfriend came a new group of "friends": brief relationships and connections made from social circles. My first big lesson in high school was not truly understanding the value of my grade school friendships that I had left behind for my new boyfriends. And the role I played in these new friend groups always seemed to be the same: I was the energy, the one who brought everyone together, the one with the ideas of fun adventures and things to do and conquer. I felt special because of this role. And when the role served its time, and the ideas ran dry, or when I realized I was again pretending to be the right fit, it would be time to move on. I would bounce to another boy and friend group, hoping that I would be liked and, in my mind, accepted.

Any crush I had I ended up "dating." Now, dating would usually only last all of a month or maybe two. One "boyfriend" I had only lasted a class period. To the high school public, a "real" boyfriend meant dating for two months. Thus, my first "real" high school dating relationship began at the end of September at the famous community Fall Fair. The boy asked me out on the Ferris wheel. That night we held hands, walked around as a new couple, and made out under the bleachers of the truck pull and derby exhibition. I had no idea at the time that this boy would be the one who would be my first partner in so many ways. He would also be my first real heartbreak and the first one to call me a slut to my face. What started off as butterflies in my stomach and head-over-heels infatuation ended in total despair, the loss of my innocence, and a ruined reputation.

The dating game was also notorious for creating drama between friends. Girls would cut you out of their friend circle if you posed a threat to one of the other girls. Everyone was quick to judge and slow to forgive. Navigating yourself through these friendships was like being on the water. Some days the sky was blue, the sun was out, and the water was calm, peaceful, and enjoyable. Other days, you braced yourself for the storm: big waves, angry water, and high drama.

My crew of girls was forever changing. The common pattern was set: the crew was a priority until a boy came on scene. As soon as a friend had a boyfriend, the crew became nonexistent unless she needed something. I was guilty of this behavior too. But the alliance of my girlfriends was mostly supportive. They would talk me through relationships and have my back. And as soon as the short-lived relationship with the boyfriends would end, I would return to the crew and act as though nothing had happened.

Any conflict that happened within the crew also had a pattern worth noticing. Conflict resolution was nonexistent. No one knew how to handle a heart-to-heart conversation or a clearing of an issue. No one addressed issues face-to-face. Instead, the girls gossiped and talked about issues behind one another's backs. We talked about each other and not to one another.

Summer came and left, along with my tan. Soon I was walking into grade ten with the hope for a better start and a better year. My grade nine year, like so many others, had been a whirlwind that left some bruises and big life lessons. Hope, which was stronger than fear, caused me to decide to move my locker down near the gym and closer to the science classrooms. The idea was to be far away from the drama and closer to a more mature crowd of people.

My breath of fresh air came when I turned my head up and was introduced to Spencer, whose locker was right beside mine. Tall with spikey blond hair and bright blue eyes, Spencer smiled at me, and all the movement in my world changed. He was my knight in a blue jacket.

My happiness and smile grew with our natural chemistry and connection. We'd sit at lunch, chatting, laughing, and flirting. We had a couple classes together, and since our lockers were beside each other, it was a run to see who got there first. Thanks to my growing relationship with Spencer, the winter season brought a flash freeze to the name calling, backstabbing, and straight-up asshole behaviors of high school pettiness. One high school dance, one kiss from the right boy, and I rose in the social graces as the girl who stole the heart of one of the princes from the hockey team.

Spencer and I started dating after that dance. I spent my weekends watching his games and attending amazing after-parties. I soon had a new crew of friendships, one that included the other girlfriends of the hockey players. Finally, things were changing for me. I started taking better care of myself, and I even stopped biting my nails, a horrible habit that I'd had since childhood. I wanted nice nails for when the time came to meet his mom. A silly idea, but hey, it worked.

Spencer and I survived the rest of the year and our long-distance summer vacation. Upon entering the beginning of grade 11, the news came that Spencer had been scouted and was moving up to the next level in hockey, the Ontario Hockey League. Although I was thrilled for him, I questioned what would happen when we were five hours apart and separated for longer periods of time. I called bullshit on the saying, "Distance makes the heart grow fonder."

With this news, things began to get strained between us, but we gave our long-distance relationship our version of our best. We made phone dates and scheduled visits for all the close games and as many weekends as we could. Then, for one game before the Christmas holidays, I decided to attend with my mom. Post game, while waiting for Spencer, my mom and I noticed a pack of girls huddled nearby glaring at me. It was awkward. We got the feeling that my name was being spoken, then fully understood why within seconds of Spencer's appearance. He came over, greeted his family and my mom, then gave me a polite kiss on the cheek. Without skipping a beat, he walked straight over to one of the girls in the pack and gave her the biggest, grossest make-out kiss ever, directly in front of us.

I couldn't move. I didn't speak, and with one look at my mom, my eyes started to well up and I nodded. It was time to go. Not fully able to process the change of events in front of me, I said my goodbyes. My mom took my hand, and with a gentle pull, we walked away. I turned back once, made eye contact with him, and in that moment, my heart broke into a million pieces. He'd clearly made his choice, and I was not it.

Telling one friend is like telling everyone in high school, especially if you don't really know who your true friends are. There I was, a topic of conversation and now, newly single. The pain I was feeling quickly turned to anger and resentment. I was at an all-time low. I wanted to stop the world and crawl into a hole.

Spencer called and called, offering up excuses and reasons for why he'd cheated. Admittedly, I fought at first and wavered over whether to try again. But the more I heard him explain, the more

I sunk into a deeper level of heartache. Everything was all about him and it made me sick.

After that, I had zero capacity for bullshit high school drama. Backstabbing, gossiping, and boy issues—I hated it all. I was only three years into high school and I had far surpassed all levels and degrees of catty behavior and had witnessed so many girls get ripped apart because of it. I felt hardened by my three years and inadvertently, I developed a bulletproof shell. A toughness.

HERstory

MEGAN

"As a competitive figure skater, I knew dedication, long hours, and practice on and off the ice, but when my mom's cancer nearly took her life, everything changed. It's funny what you take refuge in. My switch to hockey became my place of safety, support, play, and belonging. I found my people. For a teenage girl not living in the teenage world, that was everything."

A watershed moment is a turning point, the exact moment that changes the direction of an activity or situation; a dividing point from which things will never be the same. A watershed moment in a person's life has the power to completely change everything in and of their world, including themselves.

When a moment of this magnitude occurs during our younger adolescent years, it can become an ingrained memory that has lasting effects on a person's development, their identity, their sense of self, their direction, and how they navigate through the world.

It is also often recognized in hindsight. To an adolescent, these concepts can be hard to grasp.

Megan recalls the watershed moment when her world completely changed at age ten, and in that shift, she was no longer a young child but a responsible, overly careful, and perfectionistic adolescent. What helped her, however, was the friendships she found with a team of girls.

Megan had known that her mother was unwell, but her sickly behaviors were noted as unexplained. Megan, her younger brother, and their father had no idea the severity of her sickness until they experienced the mad dash to the hospital after she collapsed in their kitchen. Shortly after their arrival, Megan's mother underwent emergency surgery to save her life. While at their family friend's house, in all of a matter of hours, Megan understood that nothing was going to be the same.

In the waiting room, the Bermuda Triangle of hospitals where time stands still and everything moves in slow motion, Megan's father waited to hear the results and causes of his wife's downturn. From there, he would relay the information to Megan and her brother. It was stage III low grade non-Hodgkin lymphoma.

To Megan, her mother was a strong-willed woman who, in that period of Megan's life, she did not have the most connected relationship with. Megan said, "She was hard and quick to anger—a very strong person. She had high expectations of herself and those around her. The bar was always set high for her, right from the beginning of her life. She was also a fighter and was not going to back down to any form of cancer or its death threats."

News of this gravity is difficult for everyone connected to the patient. Megan knew something was wrong when her father invited her to go for a drive to get hot chocolate. It was his "calling card" for difficult times. Sitting in the passenger seat, Megan learned the weight of the situation.

To Megan, processing the information felt surreal; it felt unreal and difficult to comprehend. It wasn't until the symptoms and side effects appeared and her mother's appearance started to change that the gravity of it all sunk in and the fear of judgment began lurking. For Megan, her mother's hair loss was the most upsetting, as now everyone was going to know that her mom was sick and that they were different. Their world would be a topic of conversation. Everything would be visible, and thus, real.

At school, Megan's friends could not understand how Megan was feeling. They thought it was "super cool" that her mother wore all different styles of fashionable wigs. Megan's mom picked wigs to match her mood and how she was feeling that day. To try to explain to her friends that the wigs were there to cover up her bald head and sickness was frightening, and she started to feel isolated and alone.

Megan, being a witness to her mother's treatment, symptoms, and side effects, tried her best to keep her life intact and everything within the home flowing and at ease. Outside of school, she was a competitive figure skater. She had a rigorous practice schedule several times a week; something that some of her friends did not understand or participate in. At home, Megan was the one doing the laundry, making the lunches for herself and her brother, organizing playdates for him, doing the cooking, and writing the school notes. Through this change, Megan became shy, quiet, and reserved, as well as overly aware and cautious about everything. She receded.

Megan's report card home was a warning sign to her parents. One comment became the watershed moment of their daughter. It read: "Fearful that Megan is going to have a mental breakdown." Additionally, Megan's controlled behavior and her perfectionistic tendencies were becoming alarming to her father. There was no joy in Megan, no spark or happiness. Everything was serious, including skating.

To Megan, however, she was making her parents' life easier by working so hard at everything she did at home, in school, and at figure skating. She was even keeping the peace in the family and protecting / caring for her brother. Megan was content when she knew she was helping her dad manage everything while her mom put her time, energy, and effort into not dying.

But the red flags were there. Her dad, worried about Megan's mental decline, spoke up. He saw a sign at the community rink, advertising a new girls hockey league. Seeing an opportunity for his daughter, he reached out to other dads and convinced them to make the switch from figure skating to girls' hockey.

Megan could skate and introducing her to the foundations of hockey and teamwork would hopefully bring joy back to her life. Soon after, Megan, along with a couple girls she knew from skating, joined the girls' hockey league.

Unlike with girls at school, Megan had found her team in hockey. They welcomed her in and showed her how to play. When they won, they celebrated. When they lost, they had each other to lean on. The locker room became a place of connection. Megan felt the love of a team and had a place where she belonged. These girls were her support system.

Conversations about the game also translated into real-life lessons for Megan. The social language of dreams, big visions, teamwork, and encouragement, plus the competitive nature of the sport, all spoke to her. In hockey, Megan could breathe. She found her feet back on the ice, a spark in her soul, and the safety that she craved. It eased her stress. As her mom's health improved, she too found her own joy and happiness. Simultaneously, they began to heal.

For Megan, the arena and the game of hockey gave her a sense of community and the friends she'd longed for. She looked forward to practicing and getting involved in her life, both on and off the ice. She felt a renewed sense of being a kid again. An evolution had happened; something beautiful had come out of something so dark. In finding the people who supported her, Megan's inner confidence grew, she regained strength, and her happiness returned.

BARBARA

"No one was coming to save me. I had to do that by myself. I had my back and would make it through this. I needed a hero, so I became one for myself."

The journey from vulnerability to courage first starts with the confidence to be vulnerable. Our personal armor is created when we struggle with the aftermath of an event(s) in our life that inflict pain or do harm. The armor acts as a barrier, protecting our most cherished and sacred source— our inner being, our heart. To break down or dismantle the armor, one must find the power within themselves, the inner confidence to go through the pain, in order to unearth the vulnerability and find the courage to release it. It is the act of replacing the armor with the hero's cape—in finding our superhuman or heroine strength—that power resides.

Barbara entered grade ten believing it to be an opportunity for recreating herself; it was an opportunity to set in motion a new version of Barbara. Grade nine had been experimental. Figuring out the whole "dating" thing and what is acceptable and what is not is confusing for any young girl, and Barbara and her friends had been no exception. But grade ten would be different.

One night, Barbara, together with her two best friends, had plans to attend the huge house party of a mutual friend. It was a moving party, so the house was completely empty. Walking through crowds of people, the three girls who arrived together became separated. Barbara had no idea where her friends had gone. One minute they'd been together laughing, and the next, she was searching for them.

Barbara saw familiar faces, people she socialized with and friends in her classes, and she stopped to chat but didn't care about the conversations. She was focused on asking if anyone had seen her friends. No one answered, no one offered any help, so she continued walking in zigzags, feeling lost and disconnected.

Like a deer walking in an open field in fall, Barbara was vulnerable to predators. Two boys noticed Barbara's isolation and inability to speak coherently. They told her that they knew where her friends were and to follow them. "They are just down the street at another party. Come, we will take you there," she remembers them saying.

Barbara's intuition kicked in while walking down the street with them. She noticed the streetlights and was aware that they were heading in the wrong direction. She stopped and tried to turn back, but the boys, sly and full of reassurance, told her that they would find her friends soon and to keep following them.

They stopped by a field across from the high school. Barbara could see the track and the scoreboard, the library entrance and the parking lot. She had watched football games there and had run track and field activities. Barbara knew where she was but not who she was with. For a moment, she turned her head away and felt the nudge to leave. Instead of following that nudge, though, she headed straight into the point of no return and followed the boys onto the field where she was forced onto her hands and knees in the dirt. There, the boys took what wasn't theirs to take, stood up, laughed, and left her in the dark, a bloody, bruised, and disoriented mess. In state of fear and shock, Barbara felt as though she detached herself from her body, from herself. After staring at the streetlights for a while, she got off the ground slowly, brushed the dirt from her clothes, and headed back to find her friends. They were her safety. They would help.

Upon her return to the party, she was stopped by a close male friend who asked if she was okay. He had noticed her absence and told her that her mother had come and picked up one of her friends. Intent on finding the other friend, Barbara insisted she was okay and refocused her energies. Suddenly Barbara heard fighting coming from upstairs where the hosts of the party were arguing about calling the cops and an ambulance over the state that Barbara's friend was in. Puke was everywhere, and she was lying in the middle of it looking lifeless.

Barbara let out a gut-wrenching roar—a sound that had not come out when she needed to protect herself just minutes before. She realized that while she had been unable to help herself, she could and would protect and defend her friend. Barbara dragged her out of the vomit, cleaned her up, then found a place of refuge. They hid from the cops in a nearby closet.

Barbara knew what had happened to her in that field, but at that moment, she could not process it. Instead, she focused on protecting her friend as a way of protecting herself. With a task at hand, Barbara released the panic that was building up in her. It helped her settle, but it also made her suppress what had happened.

Morning light came, and carrying her friend up to her front door and into her mom's care was the first of many walks of shame Barbara had to face after that night. She knew her friend's mom was beyond furious with Barbara, and the blame was put on her shoulders. Barbara heard every harsh word of disappointment, but she didn't let the words or her feelings penetrate the shield she had now wrapped around herself.

Returning home, Barbara, still in a haze, showered off the dirt, washed away the evidence, and covered her body and bruises. Darkening her room with curtains, she laid in her bed, closed her eyes, and watched the replay of her whole night over and over and over while silently crying.

"I was alone in every sense of the word. Who could I tell? What should I do? How would I get to the doctor's office? What is Plan B, and is that the right step? How do I tell my boyfriend and friends? How do I process what's just happened to me? Who do I turn to?"

Barbara was flooded with questions, confusion, and overwhelming feelings. In looking for answers, she recognized that she had her own back and although alone on this journey, she would protect herself from everyone and anything that was coming her way. She was the injured animal, backed up in a corner, and her only way out was through.

It all began soon enough. That Sunday—the longest yet shortest day of her life—she took a late-night phone call. Her sweet, funny, heart-led, guitar-playing boyfriend was calling, demanding to know why his girlfriend had cheated on him. The rumor was out.

She tried to tell him through her tears that he didn't understand, that he had it all wrong. She hadn't betrayed him. But he would have none of it. He was hurt, lashing out, and protecting his own heart. As his upset turned to embarrassment, he broke up with her right there without hearing her speak.

The next morning, with bags under her eyes, a body covered in bruises, and her head hanging low, Barbara prepared herself to enter her morning class. She was greeted with a song, a chant on repeat: "Slut! Whore!" Like all good gossip, word had spread throughout the high school, the small town, and the neighboring towns. "Barbara, the town slut who takes two guys at a time, is single and open for business."

Judgment came from all directions and without warning. Girls took aim and demolished her with their words, dirty looks, and name calling, banishing her from all social graces. Her reputation was ruined, wrecked, and pulverized, as was her self-worth. There was no place to hide; there was no place safe for retreat. Even her own crew of girls no longer wanted her around.

"The boys wanted one thing from me: sex. I was worthless for anything else. But the girls, they were ruthless. I was conflicted. What was more destructive? Being raped or the way that these girlfriends, and girls who didn't even know me, treated me? I was washed-up trash and thrown away. And it didn't stop with just the high school girls. That afternoon, after surviving the day at high school, all I wanted was to be held by my family, to be safe in their arms. All I needed was support and protection, but what I got broke my soul. I was an embarrassment to my family, to my father's good name. I lost my mom's support and approval. I was shamed, yelled at, and blamed for a crime I didn't commit. I was not a slut, I was raped, and now I felt unworthy of a voice, unworthy of love, protection, and safety. No one was coming to save me. I had to do that by myself. I needed a hero, so I became one."

Barbara's experience of being raped, shamed, and outcast was just the beginning for her. Her trip to the pharmacist for Plan B followed by days, weeks, and months of bullying and years of being called a slut did not compare to the sister wounds that landed deep within her. Her heart shattered more from the girls' removal of sisterhood comfort and safety than her body being bruised by the act of rape.

Barbara's traumas led to her creating a fortress so tall, strong, and indestructible that she soon understood the feelings of power and powerlessness. Her backbone, self-armor, and defenses grew in strength. The silencing of her true story ate away her trust in people. She could not go back and change what happened to her; it was now a piece of her history. Barbara felt the gravity of the experience in every way and instead of remaining in the deep with it, she chose to suppress the event as an initial way to find comfort and relief.

It wasn't until many years later while Barbara was in university studying human psychology and sociology that the feelings about the experience resurfaced. This time, Barbara found solace in knowledge and in resources. She first opened up to her best friend, then her boyfriend. And as a way to regain her power, she began studying the signs and symptoms of and healing practices for sexual assault. Knowledge is power.

With her newfound knowledge combined with the powerful influences from Barbara's relationships with strong female role models, mentors, and educators in her university classes, she gradually released the hold of the fear and pain and replaced it with love and admiration for her new sisterhood. As she softened, she became aware of other young girls and women who wore the same bruises and fought similar wars. One early morning, a "sister" woke her up in need of help for she too was a victim of sexual assault. Barbara was keen to help. She knew what to do, where to go, and how to be there for HER. Barbara didn't flinch. She trusted herself and was confident that she could make a difference for the woman.

Barbara's new secret weapon was her ability to find love within herself and her sisterhood. She developed an intuitive nudge, a feeling and an eye for other girls and women who had experienced their own level of betrayal, hurt, and anguish caused by the savage act of assault and the destruction of sister wounds. She heard it in their stories and saw it in responses in social settings. Barbara, now fueled with support systems, knowledge, resources, and a passion to help, let down her guard. Although she had worn her scars of being raped in secret, she grew in strength by helping others find their way. She worked discretely, drove them to help centers, held them while they cried, and stood up and defended them against the gossipers and name callers. She became the hero that she needed, just without the cape.

YOURstory

The power of influence during the transitional period of adolescence is huge. Peer pressure, fitting in, social media, and what feels like a million expectations and "don't dos" can really take their toll on young adults. Support systems within your peer groups, friendships, mentors, coaches, and family are incredibly important. Equally important is one's ability to look out for others as well as themselves.

REFLECTION:

Look back at your younger years and identify who showed up for you through good times and bad. How did that make you feel? In what ways did YOU show up for others? For yourself? How did those relationships change and/or impact your world?

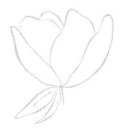

Chapter 4:
Being Labeled and the Power of Knowledge

In the last couple months of grade eleven, with absolutely zero interest in or desire to start dating or even commit any more of my time to a boy, I focused all my attention on much bigger goals and ambitions: ME! I wanted more from the town I lived in and the people who surrounded me. My version of more became less about other people and more about myself, so I invested my time into thoughts of my future and where I wanted to go.

Guidance counselors and homeroom teachers had started preparing us for our next steps. They wanted to make sure that our plans for college, university, and the employment world were set. I had always known that I wanted to be a primary/junior teacher. My goals were to complete my education and make all the necessary changes needed to finally help the children who fell through the system's cracks, simply because they didn't learn like everyone else. Students like my brother and me. As I child, I had always wanted to be smart. I wanted my voice heard and to be taken seriously, but up until grade seven and eight, teachers labeled me "slow," something that completely shut me down as a student.

Most of my early teachers reported that I lacked the ability to read, write, or compute at grade level. My grade four teacher "saw" me, though. She believed in my abilities and pushed me to see them as well, but it wasn't until I entered grade eight that I truly found my stride in academics. Mr. Williams changed things for me. He offered me the opportunity to get the direct instruction I needed. My marks came up because he believed in me, and for the first time, I believed in me too. I told Mr. Williams about my goal of getting honors by the end of the year. A simple high five cemented the challenge.

After months of dedicating myself to my homework, I got the payoff at the grade eight graduation. Mr. Williams called my name to receive my diploma, and yes, I had indeed earned honors and was even awarded the most improved student of the year. Tears rolled down my cheeks. I had done it! ME! It was my hard work, my dedication. It was all my extra hours studying and asking for additional help. I'd skipped doing the dishes numerous times just so I could reach this goal and prove to myself and all the teachers who said I wouldn't achieve anything that I could. I was proud of ME. I stood tall in my red graduation dress and was ready to show everyone I was brave, bold, a whole lot of "too much," and now, smart too! I dared to lead and was fierce and fearless. I was everything I wanted to be.

As I prepared for my last years in high school and for my future, my goal was to be the leader for change that would help every student excel. I selected my next course load, wrote my exams for the year, and left school behind for a much-needed summer holiday.

That summer was one of fun! I worked at our local provincial park as a gate girl, a job that did not require much thought. My days were simple, the sun was hot, and spending time with my girlfriends was my only priority. We took every advantage to play, enjoy the water, and get as far away as possible from anything high school related. Most of the people I was working with were older, in university, and/or not from my high school. They were refreshing to be around. Summer beach parties, no rules, just go! I felt a little rebellious that summer and loved every second of it.

With a vague understanding that there is a reason for everything, I let go of my ideals for romance and relationships. When it comes to lessons of the heart, we may not be aware enough to see everything work itself out. Whether it is insight or foresight, when it is time for you to see the lesson, that is when the next door of opportunity opens, and your heart along with it.

For me, my heart opened when I met Darryl.

Soon enough we were rounding the end of summer and September was hovering. The staff summer-end party information was posted on the board. Our park was hosting a volleyball tournament and summer bonfire, and we asked the neighboring parks to join. I had no interest in playing, but watching the game and attending the party? That was a solid yes.

That evening I sat on the boardwalk with a couple girls I worked with; we were in the prime location to watch our park team play its final game. The sun was still hot and glowing, and right before my eyes, he was there! Golden tan, blond hair, blue eyes, strong, he hit a powerful strike. It was a straight-out-of-a-movie kind of moment. I pulled down my sunglasses for a better look and asked the girls, "Who is that?"

"Oh, that's Scoob!"

"Who?"

Laughing, I asked for clarification. His name was Darryl but apparently everyone and their mother called him "Scoob." Before they could tell me anything more, I told my friends that they had to introduce me. There was something about him that had caught my eye, and I was determined to meet him. So when the game finished, we casually walked over, playing it cool, of course.

The girls introduced us and I asked him if he was planning on attending the night's bonfire and party. When he said yes, I had butterflies throughout my whole body, a reaction I had not experienced in a long time. As we left the beach to get ready and pick up our supplies for the night, I was full of excitement, almost giddy. He would be at the party; my summer was now complete.

My anticipation grew as I waited for him to arrive. He came late, but oh what an arrival. When Darryl finally made his appearance, my heart skipped a beat. He walked smoothly through the crowd, saying his hellos and giving high fives for the volleyball victory. He then headed straight toward the empty seat right beside me, which I had intentionally put there and saved just for him. We sat under the stars in the light of the bonfire, and although there was a huge party happening around us and people wanting our attention, we never broke conversation. Our focus was on each other. He made me laugh and was full of topics to talk about and stories to share. I felt at ease and as light as air.

Darryl and I went to two different high schools, something that I actually appreciated, as it allowed me to focus the next two years on reaching my goals. I wanted to spend my final years of high school improving my grades, gaining work experience to add to my résumé, and preparing for university applications. I wanted to be the first one in my family to go to university.

Everything about Darryl was smooth. He had it all and did it all. A total package. He was top of his class in academics, had big goals of attending university to become a doctor, was an all-around competitive athlete, and was liked by absolutely everyone. And then, there was me.

I was still feeling bruised and banged up from my previous relationship. I started to question how everything came to be and why. Why did he want to date me? What was attracting him to me? At that time, I had not heard of self-fulfilling prophecies, self-sabotage, or impostor syndrome, but I had witnessed these things in many of my girlfriends' relationships. We had all questioned our worth at some time or another, especially in comparing ourselves with other girls. Little did I know then, though, that I would check off each of these things at the beginning of this new, bright, and happy relationship. But Darryl and I took our time building a connection, something that slowly helped grow my confidence in myself and us.

We both had very clear directions and career paths in mind. Darryl applied to the universities that had the best health sciences programs, and I applied to art/science, concurrent education.

There was only a small handful of schools that offered both, so we knew we had to have the conversation about the possibility that we would not be attending the same school and what that would mean for our relationship. The topic of long distance was definitely a sore spot for me.

Darryl received his acceptance letter to McMaster University in Hamilton, Ontario. It was the acceptance he had really wanted to get. We had toured the school together, and as I watched him light up during the tour, I knew that that was where he would be going. And just a couple days after Darryl's letter arrived, I got my offer package from Nipissing University in North Bay, Ontario, and knew my world was about to change. I ran to my dad's office screaming, "I GOT IT! Holy shit, Dad, I did it!"

And I had. I was the one who had improved my marks, earned the requirements, and was accepted into both my undergraduate degree program and the concurrent education one. Nipissing was the school to go to if you wanted to be a teacher, and I'd be there. I was accepted!

After all the jumping and excitement, reality set in. Darryl had accepted McMaster's offer, and if I accepted at Nipissing, we would be eight-plus hours away from each other for a four-year period. So I hesitated in fear of what I might lose. My dad stepped in and gave me his form of tough love. He reminded me of my goals, my dreams, and my desires to change the world as a teacher, and I accepted the offer at Nipissing. It was what I wanted and what I had earned.

Darryl and I, although excited for each other, were also heavy-hearted knowing the distance that our education dreams would cause us. Come September, we would embark upon the challenges of long distance. Making our peace with this decision did not come without worries, insecurities, and doubt. I was thankful to have supportive parents and friends talk me through everything. Feeling more settled about my decision with Nipissing, I went to check the mail one more time.

Divine timing is a trickster.

Not even a week after sending off my acceptance letter to Nipissing, I got an acceptance package from McMaster University. But everything was already done: my paperwork and tuition checks had already been submitted. I could not go back and change it, nor would my father allow me to. Besides that, I had overcome the label of "slow" and had been accepted to my school of choice. So countdown to long distance was on: we had four months to prepare and enjoy time together.

HERstory

ALICIA

"I remember walking home from school with other kids, listening to them talk about home and school and how they were dealing with their own lives. One of the girls said to me in front of the group, 'You wouldn't understand because you are perfect.' Her point of view stopped me. Inside, my inner voice started to scream, *If I am not perfect, then something bad is going to happen.* This was the jump-off mark that took me on a journey of control."

According to Simply Psychology, labeling theory is a concept that focuses on the ways in which influential people, peers, family/friends, guides, teachers—the agents of change in people's worlds—attach a stereotype to a person and/or group. What happens next is that the stigmatized person/people change their behavior to reflect the labeled stereotype.

For example, if someone is told over and over that they are stupid, they will internalize it and start behaving stupidly. They take on the characteristics, the persona, the behaviors of the deviant label—the judgment. Labeling theory is linked to self-fulfilling prophecies.

In high school, Alicia was a committed student and athlete, belonged to the "popular" group, was a high achiever, and was kind and seemingly confident. She was labeled *perfect* by her peers, teachers, coaches, family, friends, and parents.

To Alicia, though, her high school years brought out two different versions of her: the socially labeled "perfect" girl that everyone knew, and the troubled and conflicted girl that was looking back at her in the mirror. Due to labeling, the word *perfect* ran on repeat in her mind and soon became all-encompassing. As a result, Alicia became self-conscious and believed she couldn't let herself do anything unless it was done absolutely perfectly. To the outside world, Alicia was fine. Internally, however, Alicia was battling the self-talk of unworthiness, belittlement, and defeat. Her inner voice spoke words of food control and suicide; it questioned whether the world would notice or care if she were gone.

But why was she in such a dark place? To her, it was inherited sadness. Her parents were having marital problems and brought tension into their home, and her brother was occupied by his own world. Alicia became a buffer to everyone's problems; she was a "perfect" daughter and person to offload on.

"Be perfect, be in control, and be small. I was put into a role that was chosen for me and that was not what I wanted. I needed to carry the load of school, being involved in sports, and working several jobs; plus, I had to carry the family load, which was the heaviest. It was my self-appointed job to make everything right. To me, I was born as the *peacemaker*—the fixer. I didn't want to be the strong one all the time. So, if I wasn't going to kill myself, then I would make myself so small that no one would notice me."

By grade twelve, Alicia had developed tips and tricks for hiding her real feelings. She was also incredibly observant and had picked up on other girls within her circle who were hiding similar secrets. Alicia was definitely not the only girl experiencing sadness, depression, and acts of self-harm.

At the time, Alicia was in denial that she was depressed and that anyone had any idea about the gravity of her illness. She thought she was getting away with it all. From this place, her deep-seated feelings plus the "perfect" social portrait landed heavily on her life. What was building inside of her was her need to control everything, and specifically, food. Her feelings of sadness led to the desire to feel "empty." From there, she found a way to curb her appetite to keep the emptiness satisfied.

Alicia kept herself busy with schoolwork and extracurricular activities, hoping no one would notice how much she was limiting herself. She told her parents that she was trying to be "healthy." By her final year of high school, her daily routine was systematic. She had gotten a membership at a local gym where she exercised every morning before school, then at night, she exercised at home in her room. This routine, plus her limited calorie intake, slowly ate away at her body until the light in her eyes dimmed.

"On the outside, I had it all together and was thriving. People were telling me how great I looked. My grades did not falter, my job performance and athletic pursuits continued, and my closet behavior went untouched. But my eyes said it all. I had dead eyes."

Friday would roll around, the weekend parties would begin, and Alicia's sense of control would release with every sip of lemon gin she consumed. The bottles would stack up, the munchies would come out, and Alicia would be "free" from the constraints of her weekly diet. She ate, drank, and ate some more—until Sunday morning arrived with a guilt trip. Panic would set in, and Alicia would become consumed with disgust. She'd then force herself to throw up all the evidence and return to the state of emptiness.

Her closest friends witnessed it all—they watched Alicia party to the point of blackout on weekends and then clean up in time for Monday morning classes. As much as they were witnesses, they, too, were struggling alongside her. Alicia knew of four other girls in her grade who were "secretly" anorexic and others who struggled with alcoholism. Although they were in the same social circle, no one spoke about it.

When an older girl at Alicia's school died of anorexia, Alicia's secret life began to unravel. As the community mourned, Alicia's brother came to her room one night in tears. He asked, "Are you going to die too?" That night, afraid of losing his sister, he slept on the floor beside her. Her secret was out. People close to her were starting to figure it out.

Alicia's parents were next. They confronted her and challenged her to eat a bagel in front of them. Alicia was paralyzed with fear and could not take one bite. From there, they insisted that she go to a clinic in a nearby town to determine her mental state and the severity of her "problem." The clinic staff interviewed her, but unfortunately, they didn't recognize how ill Alicia really was and deemed her "not sick enough" to start any treatment strategies or plans.

Life continued. Alicia was dating a boy, her schoolwork still earned her top grades, and she adjusted back into her weekday controlled and disordered eating and weekend partying. She continued to hide her behavior until her boyfriend caught her purging one night after dinner. He expressed his concerns and how fearful he was for her, and things started to crumble. First the death of an older girl with a similar illness, then her family's concerns, and now her boyfriend. Alicia started to realize for herself how far down this path she'd gone. Her image of perfection had to go. Her darkness was showing its face as a form of depression that was finally being identified and named.

But Alicia's cycle of control, her embedded fear of the lack thereof, and the role being anorexic played in obtaining that sense of control followed Alicia into her next phases of life. She saw the severity of her situation and her declining health, but it did not result in a lightbulb moment for change. It took several moments and time to pile up for the cycle to be disrupted.

The silence of these struggles that surrounded Alicia and her friends needed to be broken, and she knew it. Each of them, dealing with their own self-destructive behaviors, needed similar support and a voice to share their stories. Understanding this need for herself and for them, Alicia felt the strong nudge and sense of purpose change her course, a trajectory that would point Alicia in the direction of studying human biology and women's health in university. Alicia fell in love with gathering knowledge about how the female body works and operates. Inadvertently, she fell in love with the idea that this knowledge could impact other women as well, and she may be able to save them too.

Confident and lit up by the challenge of learning more, finding help, and being a voice for the silent, Alicia's purpose to help and save others would be discovered when she ultimately decided to BE the impact; and to her, that meant living.

BRITTANY

The captain of both her soccer teams—high school and elite—Brittany loved the support and cushion of friends and family that came with it. She had all the confidence in the world. She knew who she was and what her drive, ambition, athleticism, and work ethic could award her. She was on her way to the big leagues: she had a chance to be scouted for scholarships to the States.

Right before her departure, she experienced an athlete's worst nightmare of an injury. While lingering in the unknown for about a year after the first real blow to her confidence and her goals in life, Brittany, now a freshman in her first year of university, experienced a second hit with the unexpected death of a friend.

The shifts came with a new perspective and left Brittany confused. She hadn't yet established friendships, she had no team to belong to, she was in a new city, and she was experiencing the layers of grief that came from mourning her friend and her old life. Questions like "Who am I?" left Brittany feeling a new level of low.

Dorm-style residency had opened Brittany's world up to a melting pot of new people—people who did not seem to even notice she was there. She would say hello and extend a friendly greeting with the hope of making connections, only to be met with dirty looks and people passing her by. Brittany felt foreign, outcast. She was disconnected and not sturdy on her feet.

Second semester, Brittany transferred to a different university for a fresh start. Her new focus was on taking this opportunity to get back to her normal routine, which meant working out and being social. The gym was like a second home to her. This is where she would meet her people—other athletes.

The relationships she was forming and the sturdiness of her long-term boyfriend were refreshing at first. But in a short period of time, the teeter-totter effect appeared. Brittany experienced yet another major health crisis within her family, her friend circle began changing, and her relationship took a turn for the worse, so she ended it. As a result of these crises, Brittany turtled. There was no safe place to seek comfort. She became uncomfortable in her own skin, and her self-image took a hit.

Brittany needed to find some solid ground and get structure back in her world. With her new goal of focusing on herself, she started to omit certain types of foods that were under her structured diet plan. The idea was to keep her athletic build and to reduce weight. The goal was to lose only five to ten pounds. Little did she realize that the lack of substantial food would deplete her and that some of her food choices caused an allergic reaction in her body. She began having feelings of failure, and she couldn't commit to or complete a program like she once had. The allergic reactions she was experiencing caused Brittany to vomit, and now, to replace the feelings of failure, throwing up became her new stress release.

Instead of dealing with the pain and other emotions she was suffering from, Brittany filled her time with daily trips to the gym, schoolwork, and mental notes of the "good" food and "bad" food she ate. Before long, she realized she couldn't stop the controlled behavior. She had become addicted to the release, the emptiness, and the shame.

"Before I realized what I was going through, I paused and reflected back to the time when I was a part of a team and believed I would NEVER be the one who would have an eating disorder. But there I was, living off adrenaline, fear, and stress—I wasn't in my body. I was on automatic mode, and something was about to give."

By the spring of second year, she no longer recognized herself. A new fear came to the surface. Brittany fully understood she had an eating disorder. She took a deep breath and called her big brother for help; she admitted that she had a problem.

"As soon as I told him, I told someone, my disorder went into full force. I began throwing up ten times a day instead of a couple times a week. I became depressed, anxiety hit, and my body mirrored it."

Brittany was lost and in a constant state of fear and isolation. Just a mere glimpse of herself caused her to crumble to the floor in tears. She wondered what had happened to her, what had happened to the girl who once danced in the kitchen every morning. Her sense of urgency grew, and Brittany realized that she needed to focus on finding out who she would or could become.

Brittany's eating disorder took more than her external appearance and health—it took her belief in herself and her self-worth. Telling her brother had been a start, and now Brittany knew the second step would be telling her parents and seeking help from doctors. When she told her mother, her mom said, "I will let you heal your own way, but I have one ask—that you go talk to someone, a therapist."

Brittany followed her mother's request and began seeing the first therapist that was referred. Unfortunately, her therapy sessions felt like a transaction process. Brittany would be just breaking through the surface of her struggles when the therapist's timer would go off, indicating the end of the session. Brittany intuitively knew that this was not the right fit for her.

By this time, things were truly serious. Brittany's hands had turned yellow, she was constantly bloated, and she felt as if the walls to receiving the right kind of help were far too high and out of reach for her. Doctors and therapists who relied on ticking timers and poor remedies that masked symptoms for treatment plans that were not suited for her or the root causes of her problem were of no help.

With little hope, body fatigue, and a haunting fear of death settling in, Brittany went quiet. Her inner light dimmed by the day, and she began questioning the purpose of life. Thankfully, Brittany received a lifeline from a friend of the family, someone close enough to them to know what was happening to her. Brittany recalls this friend saying, "She needs to meet Joy."

"Joy is an energy healer. I was unsure of what that even meant, but I was eager to try anything. She tapped my head, my heart, and then parts of my body, all of which sparked sensations like an electric current. For the first time I had hope."

After her meeting with Joy, Brittany, on her return home, ran and slid in her socks on the hard floor toward her mom. She declared, "Mom! She is going to be the one who saves me." Her mom flooded her with questions, diving deep to understand more about what Brittany was experiencing. Brittany eased her mom's questions by saying, "I don't know, Mom, but I feel HOPE."

Brittany saw Joy once a month over the next few years. During their time together, Joy sparked Brittany's curiosity in energy healing modalities and alternative medicine. These modalities showed Brittany a new perspective that infused color back into her black-and-white world.

Joy taught Brittany how to understand her body, how energy moves, and how to use the powers of elements around and in us, all of which empowered Brittany as she gained belief in her own abilities to heal herself. She became in tune with her own body as well as how to tap into those around her. As Brittany became stronger mentally, physically, emotionally, and spiritually, she became more aware of her own curiosities and desires to study energy medicine.

Seeking more knowledge, Brittany bought a one-way ticket to Australia with the goal of discovering herself—her identity outside of the world of school, sports, and her past eating disorder. In Australia, Brittany taught her body how to heal and listen to energetic pulls and vibrations. It opened her eyes to what her happiness is—it's found deep within her own being.

YOURstory

Knowledge is power. It unlocks and sparks confidence and curiosity and opens us up to understanding new truths of the world. It can be a powerful tool for self-growth of any kind, and it can help us overcome the labels we've received. Maya Angelou, a famous author, poet, and educator, is often credited as saying, "When you know better, do better." And when you know better and do better, pass that knowing, that knowledge, on to others.

REFLECTION:

Have you ever experienced being labeled? Did it help you or hinder you? How has the power of knowledge influenced your life? Have you used that knowledge to help someone else?

Chapter 5:
Friendship, Love, and Romance

Before we knew it, the time came for Darryl and me to leave for university. As this was the first move away from our parents' homes and into a resident-style living quarters, it was a huge life event for both of us. Plus, our long-distance relationship started the second we drove off in opposite directions.

Lucky for me, my best friend, Devon, was my roommate and together, we would embark on this big moment. She was also in a long-distance relationship with her high school sweetheart, and ironically, he, too, was at McMaster University, so Devon and I had each other to take comfort in. When we finally settled into our rooms and the reality of our big move set in, we started the first big steps in our first big city.

Despite my close friendship with Devon, the shock and total life change took its toll on my emotional, physical, and mental health. Within two months, I became more reclused and withdrawn. It felt like a loss of identity. I was starting to make other friendships and get the lay of the land, but I felt distanced. I didn't jump right into the so-called university life. I lost twenty pounds from the stress of it all, plus having to meal plan, prep, and shop for all the groceries on my own for the first time. I was missing home, my parents, my brother and friends, and especially Darryl. Together they were my safety net and the comfort I felt like I needed to be myself.

Devon and I traveled together to McMaster University to visit the guys as often as we could. These visits required a lot of travel time: an eight-hour bus or train to Toronto and then a transitional stop to get the next bus to Hamilton. We often would do the red-eye trips; we'd travel during the night and arrive at McMaster by 8 a.m.

On the occasion that I took the trip solo, the sense of security I felt while traveling with Devon was sometimes replaced with fear. I was a small-town girl who was afraid of city transit, and I was now traveling alone on the red-eye bus. But these trips strengthened my independence. I figured out all the stops and transitions and always made it to Darryl's dorm. It was empowering, and it built my confidence.

Darryl and I were experiencing our fair share of relationship issues and were tested multiple times. The struggle of insecurities and fears of being cheated on were old wounds that kept showing up, and we started to doubt our ability to stay together. We tried to see each other at least one weekend a month, but the travel, the expenses, our different course loads, and then the winter road conditions lengthened our time away from each other. We were fighting more and feeling disconnected. We were frustrated, missing each other, and this long distance was killing us. Devon and her partner were experiencing it too, and they eventually broke up.

One night, Devon and I went to a bar. Devon was mourning her breakup and the drinks went down like water. I sensed that trouble would find us that night, and oh did it ever. Trouble came in the form of an older guy making far too many aggressive advances on Devon. I was standing off to the side watching it all take place, and I could feel my body start to respond. Anger pooled. Along with our core group of guy friends, I headed straight for the man, bracing myself to take him out. My mouth opened, and within a hot minute, a fight broke out—and Devon and I were right in the middle of it all.

That fight was the tipping point for my friendship with Devon. Prior to that night, we had started experiencing a disconnect. I was focused on mending and maintaining my relationship while also studying for exams, finding a house, and picking roommates for our second year. She was going through the stages of heartbreak and confusion. Then the bar fight occurred. Although we were not mad at each other per se, we were mad at so many other factors around us. Afterward, Devon and I took a break without ever saying we needed one. The summer break was coming, and my only focus was on seeing Darryl as much as possible; that, and avoiding a problem that I did not know how to face—the possible threat of hurting Devon and myself. At that time, I did not know how to have a difficult conversation or express myself.

Devon and I barely spoke that summer and when we did, there was a distance between us. We had words left unspoken and recurring anger. Then one argument changed everything for us.

We both wanted to be heard and validated, but stubbornness and a lack of patience kept us from hearing each other. Neither one of us was going to budge. We questioned each other's trust and intentions, and as a result, we broke up. Breaking up with my best friend was by far the greatest pain I had ever experienced, and I entered a whole new kind of deep mourning. We needed time and space to forgive, heal, and grow separately. I knew in my heart that our story was not complete, and after some time, we did reconnect. At that time, however, I needed to discover who I was flying solo.

My new roommates, Pam and Crystal, were already established friends. They had known each other since childhood. I was their third wheel, and in truth, I was happy to be. I could be a part of the trio when it served us, with the freedom to step out and away when it didn't. I loved their energy, their sense of togetherness. I respected it. Without formally discussing it, we established our roles in the house, and everything flowed beautifully. I had a special connection and uniquely different relationship with each of them.

Crystal sparked my happiness. She saw right down into my soul and pulled out the best of me. She was always up for an adventure and would declare MORE: more play, more fun, more snuggle time on the couch on Sundays. We were connected on so many levels. We brought out in each other our confidence, trust, and deep, heartfelt conversations about growth, personal needs, and safety.

Pam brought out my analytical side. We studied together, had conversations about grand theories, and strove for excellence in school. And on weekends we'd have forever dance parties where we really connected. We were roommates who also respected the other's search for independence. We never said we had to do absolutely everything together; we had freedom to explore other friendships, social circles, activities, and hobbies.

Living with Pam and Crystal was game changing for me. I went from being in a cocoon to becoming a butterfly. This was an impactful lesson for me about the importance of my environment and the people I surrounded myself with. I went from being a "no girl" to a "yes girl" over night. They brought play back into my life, as well as a sense of safety. We had a system, and that system supported all of us. They sparked in me in a new level of confidence. This led to me branching out and making connections with Roslyn, my partner in crime and best friend in university, plus a whole crew. These friendships I made in university became my whole world.

All the new adventures I was saying YES to we did together: Frosh leadership opportunities, exploring North Bay, cliff jumping, target practice during hunting season, winter sports, themed parties . . . and the list continues. These four years of university life were the entrance to what I refer to as the Glory Years of my life. I surrounded myself with people who loved life and went after everything they did with the intention of having the best experience ever.

School wise, I was absolutely in love with psychology, women's studies, and sociology. I found my niche. All the theories and studies and new global perspectives truly lit up my world of knowledge. I looked at the world with a new lens, and then when I refocused, I looked at people differently. I started to understand how groups and individuals worked, their dynamics. I studied label theory and realized how as a child who was labeled "slow," I, too, got caught in the web of this theory. But as much as I loved the material and was doing my best with my grades and studies, this was university. I could not fake it to make it. And I wanted to do more than just make it; I wanted to thrive at it. I challenged myself to believe in my abilities and the fact that I could achieve whatever I set my mind to.

During third year, I sought out additional help from the professor's aide in one of my psychology courses. My paper was due soon, and I needed some extra help to break through my writer's block. But instead of offering support, the aide looked right at me in total disgust and asked, "How did you even make it into university? You can't write."

Apparently, my literary skills were so bad, so grotesque, that he could barely focus, no less help me. I thought he was being a little dramatic. But sure enough, he said I would fail the paper if I submitted my work. Flashbacks to grade school, to teachers calling me "stupid," and the walk of shame up the stairs to the "slow" kids' private class all flooded back while sitting in his office that day.

In embarrassment over not knowing how to spell or use grammar and punctuation correctly, I left his office full of doubt, my head low, completely defeated. All I wanted to do was curl up into a ball and go to bed. Instead, I answered the nudge from friends to get out of my head and dance it out with a "hell ya!" What they were really doing was shaking up my perspective and pushing me back into my inner knowing that I did get into university for all the right reasons. One person's opinion wasn't going to take that away from me. I had earned my place there.

With support and a renewed sense of ease, I rewrote my entire essay. I submitted my new paper, and a couple weeks later, I received top marks for it. That night out with my friends had recentered and relaxed me enough to write a paper from a place of knowing and believing that I could.

In fourth year, I took a part-time job at a women's gym. My position was easy: sell the merchandise, sign everyone in, make sure to greet all the ladies with a warm welcome or a happy departure, plus teach three circuit training classes a week. I had amazing energy, I loved to work out, and I viewed it more as play than work. Soon, a group of women became regular attendees of my classes. Each class was forty-five minutes of pure joy and sweat.

One day during the high intensity training, I, in the most encouraging kind of way, yelled out, "Let's GO, BITCHES!" Completely shocked that I'd yelled that, I instantly stopped and prepared myself for a backlash followed by my apologies. Instead, the women roared! They loved it! From that moment on, we were a group. We even planned social outings and ladies' nights out. It was my first experience belonging to a close community of women, and after six months of connecting with them, I felt comfortable enough to ask some of them to write a reference letter for me. I needed several letters for teacher's college and my future portfolio. Without hesitation, they jumped in, wrote, and handed me a stack of letters.

These women were powerhouses. Smart, dedicated, hardworking, and full of self-love! As I guided them in class, they guided me in life lessons. I did more listening than ever before; I took in all their stories, their life experiences, their ups and the downs;

plus, I learned how they got to the top of their game—a spot that I knew I wanted to be in one day.

My boss at the gym was going through her own background issues and was not the most pleasant person to work for. Many times, she would give backhanded compliments and would glare at me. There was an underlying current happening, and I knew it all stemmed from her own issues. I had been in that position before with lots of girls and other women. It had a distinct smell of comparison, competition, and threat. As bold as I am, in one of our weekly meetings, I addressed all the ways that the center and she, as the boss, could and should start making changes that would work for the audience, our customers.

The feedback was not received well. In fact, she lost her shit and called me "cocky"—a "know it all"—and then asked me to leave. I loved working with my ladies in the classes, but with all the behind-the-scenes drama, the henhouse banter, and the "female threat" behavior, I gladly got up and walked away.

Not even two days later, my boss called me in and apologized. She said she was struggling with her boyfriend and that in truth, the suggestions I was making were amazing and that the ladies of the gym needed them. So the adjustments were made, and the whole energy of the gym became electric! And from that point on, my position leveled up. Sometimes you just have to use your voice, face difficult conversations, stand your ground, and be prepared to walk away.

In my relationship, Darryl and I were preparing for our next big leap of faith with teacher's college and med school fast approaching. It was another round of university applications, interviews, and waiting. We were finally approaching the finish line in our long-distance relationship, and I could see the end game and was ready for the last stretch. Our plan was to set up home together wherever he got his med school acceptance. There, I would then arrange my practicum placement for teacher's college. For him, though, it was the idea of finally being together in one spot that shook him up. Commitment issues surfaced. Moving in together was the next big step, and that scared him.

Darryl got his acceptance letter to Ottawa University Medical School, and I got on the computer to make the connections for my practicum. We found a place to live, and everything was coming together. I knew we were making fast decisions, especially when Darryl started acting strangely. It was a lot to process, but I didn't overthink it, as I knew we were just feeling the weight and pressures of another September coming. But then in one heated argument, Darryl revealed why he was acting so differently. He had started to question whether we should move in together; he was nervous about it all and confused about the life changes that were ahead of us.

I was furious. Although I also shared in the confusion over the changes, I was hurt. We fought. It was four years of battle wounds plus new heightened concerns about independence and whether we would still have any if we moved in together. Teacher's college and med school were approaching fast, and a new fear that our relationship coming to an end was real.

After five weeks of fighting with Darryl and going back and forth over his new issues with committing, I threw in the white flag. I was done. If he didn't know by that point, then he would never know, and that was not good enough for me. My birthday was coming up and I didn't want to fight anymore. I had fought for our relationship for four years, and now he was unsure?

My friends saw me through it all. I spoke to them tirelessly about it and their support was immeasurable. So, after many conversations with friends and right before my birthday party, I called Darryl and ended things. I told him that he'd had all the time in the world to figure things out but that I was no longer waiting. He was upset and asked me to reconsider and give him more time to think. Out of rage, I responded, "I gave you four years."

With Darryl and me on a break, my friendships with my original university friends shifted too. I did not have my feet on the ground. It was more like a spin and in every direction. For the first time in years, I was single. It was the oddest feeling: no connections, no ties, no boundaries, no rules, nothing. I felt lost.

Meanwhile, a local election was coming up, and one of the people running for office was named Darryl, so I kept seeing "Vote for Darryl" signs everywhere I went—in elevators, on bus routes, while driving to get groceries, and all over the mall. And the music I was hearing, any and everywhere I went, consisted of our songs. Even the silly ones that were popular in the '70s and typically would not be played in malls or restaurants, bars, or in the hallways at school were playing on repeat. I brushed it all off, trying to ignore the signs to call or connect with him.

But conversations about Ottawa always circled back to Darryl and how he was adjusting to med school or my excitement about starting my placement in the capital. More times than not, everything pointed to Ottawa and to him. I wanted to respect my own boundaries with our breakup, but after a couple weeks, and a million conversations about priorities, I felt the nudge to get back in connection. On his end, he had gained all the clarity he needed. We both did.

The whole saying that "people come into your life for a reason, a season, or a lifetime" was proving its accuracy and impact during the short period of time we were apart. My transition into teacher's college introduced me to people who served the "reason." Some of the people were meant to inspire me, while others served as a reminder of a past life lesson that I'd already learned. And in my season of being single, people appeared to show me my options. They reminded me about what I loved and what I hated about the opposite sex, and what I loved about myself. Even female friendships served their season and reason. Some of my best friendships came to their end. Although at the time I did not recognize the reason or agree with their departure, it still rang true to the saying. Those relationships were meant for the university season. And then there was Darryl, the person who came into my life for a lifetime. This break was a reminder of that. I was so happy to get back together, but I was also happy that I knew more about myself.

HERstory

CASSANDRA

"I was always the single girl, the one who had a ton of amazing girlfriends who always wanted to set me up. My list of attributes for 'the man' I was going to commit to was long, and my expectations were high. On that list in bold lettering? This man would understand and honor my priorities for my lifestyle, my friendships, and my career choices, plus he would support my commitment and sacrifices to my sport. I knew the level I was playing in, and I would not settle for anyone who didn't play in it with me."

The quote "little girls with big dreams grow up to be women with big visions" is one that every little girl should hear. Let's not stop there; add to that the quote "you wouldn't have a desire or a dream unless it were within your power to make it real." When we dream big dreams, we need to know that it is in us to go after them and that they are achievable.

Little girls who watch the people in their lives, people who they deem impactful and influential, become firsthand witnesses to what commitment is, what it takes to make dreams come true, and how to live into their own power. That is the importance of role models: parents, teachers, instructors, community leaders, and grandparents.

They learn different levels of priorities and how to set them. They observe work ethics, communication, different degrees of hierarchy, and how to be seen, valued, and heard. They process how to behave, what to go after, what is and is not socially acceptable. Like little sponges, they soak up all the details about what living with and without self-worth looks like.

Cassandra, an only child, felt loved, supported, and safe from all the attention she received from her parents and grandparents. Her mother and grandmother, both professional women, were very dedicated to their own self-development, family, and community, and they instilled these values in Cassandra by leading by example.

As a competitive dancer, vocalist, and pianist, Cassandra knew all about hard work, long practices, and sacrifices. When other kids were out playing, having sleepovers, and partying as teens, Cassandra was practicing with her team and putting in the time, energy, and effort. She had goals, priorities, and big aspirations, and partying was not one of them.

Cassandra understood the level of commitment it took to turn a passion for your sport into a profession. At university, she joined the Ottawa University curling league, which propelled her interests and sparked her competitive fire of the sport.

"Joining this league brought me friendships, community, and teammates who later became sisters. It was an intimate team experience where everyone had a role, and together, we had to support each other on and off the ice. We were all going after the same goal, and because of our amazing team dynamics, we all knew that we needed to stay together to accomplish that goal."

While in university, Cassandra was known among her crew as their "single friend." Simply put, Cassandra was not interested in the dating scene, nor did she have time for all the games of the heart that came with it. She never felt as if she was missing out;

she was having lots of fun. Cassandra was an independent woman who knew what she wanted.

Career wise, Cassandra knew that she needed a profession that would mesh with her curling schedule that involved hours on the ice and traveling all over Canada. The same could be said about finding a partner in life. Cassandra knew that curling was her "baggage." The time, energy, and commitment to her teammates—she was not going to give that up for just any guy. Her sport was a huge contributor to her happiness and joy; it was not only her focus but also her priority in life.

When Cassandra joined the Ottawa Curling Club, she met many lifelong friends. She also met Gary, a man who was recently divorced and a father of two boys. At first, they only connected through their love of sport. But when she was not looking for love, love found her. She had been single for so long that this connection came unexpectedly and took her by surprise. Her list of attributes for an ideal man suddenly no longer mattered. She already knew that having children of her own was not part of her plan, so being an active part of his boys' lives was a bonus for Cassandra. She had found someone who supported her dreams and understood all the sacrifices needed to play at her current level plus the levels she was headed toward.

Gary did not want to change her world but simply be a part of it. Although there was a notable age gap between the two and outsiders looking in had their own views and comments, Cassandra and Gary passed that obstacle gracefully.

"We gave energy to ourselves, our relationship, and our love for the sport. In a long-term relationship with a partner, you travel down the road together and your priorities grow and change with you. Gary has always been my favorite person to spend time with. To me, love doesn't know circumstances, ages, or judgments. You come with your list, your deal-breakers, but when you are in it, those disappear. We face our challenges together."

Before Gary came into her life, Cassandra's first love and commitment was to herself. She was established in life with her education, team, and sport, as well as with her family and friends. Everything was a result of the fact that she knew love within herself first.

Cassandra made her life decisions for Gary, for curling, for her career, and for her role as a stepmother based on what mattered to her the most. Honoring yourself is seeing your self-worth and knowing that that is MORE than enough!

MARIE

"I'd just bought my first home all on my own. I had landed a great job in a hospital, working with a team that I adored. I was strong, independent, and happy. I will never forget the day that I met him. Soon after, I understood that life would have been better if I hadn't."

Marie grew up in a home built on love and acceptance with a strong foundation of morals, beliefs, and values. After graduating university, she was in search of her own community, partner, and a place to plant roots. She got a job at the hospital as an ultrasound technologist and saved enough to purchase her first home at age twenty-three. Shortly after, a new medical student was assigned to Marie's department.

"I was elated when he was assigned to work with me. We left the hospital together that afternoon and when he asked for my number, I had to pinch myself. We had our first date the next night and talked for hours. Things escalated quickly and I fell hard and fast. He was perfect for me. He was handsome, smart, easy to get along with, and appreciated my sense of humor. I was in love with him after a few months of dating."

It takes time to really get to know someone, to get to know who they are and what their values and beliefs are. It takes time to understand how they operate, process, handle, and deal with the twists and turns of daily life plus the grand visions of it.

Wanting to take their relationship to the next level, the man revealed his devotion to his faith and family traditions to Marie. Marie identified as atheist, but at that time, she did not fully comprehend the depth and conviction of his beliefs so didn't consider the conflict an issue. He had her heart, so she agreed to explore his belief system and values.

For the first time in her life, Marie committed to attending church every Sunday. This satisfied him for a while, but soon Marie wasn't allowed to swear or watch shows or movies that were not approved. Additionally, her friends had to be a part of the church, and all social engagements had to be within the church's boundaries. It then escalated further when her body weight, what she wore, and what she ate were monitored and controlled as well.

"He controlled everything. He said, 'I want you to fit into this dress for my graduation.' I remember that graduation. I couldn't breathe. Slowly, I became separated from my friends and family. He said that they were jealous of us and wanted what we had; that they didn't understand. I threw myself into the role he wanted me to play, the person I needed to become to be good enough. I cooked all his meals, read scripture, watched my mouth, and planned acceptable social outings with my friends from the church. Being good enough, of course, was impossible."

The holiday season arrived and so did a message from him. It took the wind right out of her and brought her to her knees. He broke up with her via text message, declaring that she wasn't faithful enough to his religion and wasn't good enough in general for him. Their relationship was over.

She never saw this breakup coming and was devastated. Her New Year's resolution was to become "enough" to win him back. She lost more weight, read more scripture and took notes, and started listening to religious music. She returned to the church with the goal of showing her devotion to him, his community, and to herself. It worked! In fact, it worked so well that he asked her for her hand in holy matrimony!

Marie's feelings of joy were short lived. Deep down in her body, in her heart and soul, she knew something wasn't right. Her discernment was firing. Once on top of the world, she was now depressed, a shell of herself; she was lost in a world of devotion to a man who was controlling her every breath. Her energy was gone, and she was no longer confident and put together. Her light had dimmed to a mere flicker, and he noticed. He retracted his proposal and put her on relationship probation. She no longer knew who she was or where she stood. She felt humiliated and degraded. She was completely powerless and at his mercy.

One year later, she received another text message that stopped everything. This time it was from her mother; it was a desperate message telling her that a family friend had died. Without questioning herself or asking for permission, Marie drove straight home. This loss was devastating to Marie's whole family; the two families had always been connected. They'd vacationed together, and their kids were like extended siblings to Marie and her sisters. It was in this heaviness that Marie came to terms with what she had become and started to wake from a horrible nightmare that was her relationship. She witnessed her parents leaning on each other in loving embraces of support and trust. Her sister's fiancé was there holding her hand, providing comfort and his heart to her and her family, including Marie.

She started to look inward and ask herself hard questions: Where was he? Why wasn't he asking how she was doing, feeling, or coping? Why wasn't he there? Upon returning home, Marie confronted him and questioned him aloud about his absence. His response was enough to push Marie into the here and now. He hadn't known the deceased, so therefore he'd decided to go cycling instead of the funeral.

It was as if a light turned on. In that moment, Marie straightened her back, grew in length, and stood strong in her values, morals, and beliefs. She asked him to leave, never to return. This time they were done, and she was the one calling it quits. He tried to regain his footing with her: he showed up unannounced; she shut the door. He called; she ignored his calls. He messaged her; she blocked him. She pushed forward and past him and never looked back.

Erasing him from her life was the hardest thing she'd ever had to do. She had to relearn who she was and to heal from the ghost-like figure she had become. She made the difficult decision to only move forward. Her motto became "blinders up and keep going."

"This relationship both consumed and destroyed me. It took all my self-confidence, my independence, and all my time. I was in too deep and thought I was in love. I was broken, and clawing out of that hole was anything but easy. The city I had come to love became toxic to me. My home felt like a prison. The hospital reeked of him. He was now a resident at the hospital I worked at which meant that avoiding him at work was impossible. I started to have extreme anxiety about running into him unexpectedly, which resulted in me having to avoid any public places. Something needed to give."

The love and support from Marie's family gave her the courage to start fresh and rebuild herself. Marie sold her house and her belongings and found a job and an apartment in a new city hours and light years away from a life she was no longer willing to live.

To start her healing, Marie first had to reclaim her power—her confidence in herself and her belief that she was more than enough. Her roots spoke loudly. With a spark of self-love and her friends' and family's devotion, acceptance, and support, Marie had the courage to take it all in, process it, and start the healing journey. With all this love, Marie gained traction in her new life and vowed to love, respect, and honor herself first. She now knows that when the true love appears, it, too, will be built on a foundation of these values.

YOURstory

The love of family, friends, and partners is wonderful, but everything changes the second you stay true to YOU. That is the art of self-love: honoring your needs, wants, and heart's desires.

To know love, it starts with you. Love yourself first, and the rest will follow.

REFLECTION:

Relationships are important, but none more than the one you have with yourself. What does self-love mean to you?

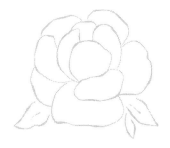

Chapter 6:
Transitions and Choices

I had arrived! Ottawa, our nation's capital, and my new home! I already loved everything about the city. It had a welcoming sense to it, and I loved the rush of the traffic and the flow. We lived a walkable distance to the canal, the market, Bank Street, and the Glebe and all its cafés and shops. It was a great location. From our apartment window, we could see Parliament, which also meant that anytime there were fireworks, we got the best view.

For Darryl and me, it was our first experience living together, and although I was only there for weeks at a time for teaching placements and we shared the space with a friend, it was a great introduction to our new commitment. After our brief breakup, we needed to work through our insecurities, rebuild trust, and figure out how to share time. We had gotten used to the formality of a long-distance relationship. This was an adjustment.

Being new to the city, I had to establish myself. I needed to figure out how to drive on the highway, find shopping places for groceries and personal needs, and make my own connections. Darryl had started making new friends within the world of med school, and I needed to meet new people and create my own friendships.

The first friend I made was Susan, whose husband was in med school with Darryl. Susan was a fellow teacher, so we had a lot in common and were working toward the same goals. Susan had her foot in the door of the school system, as she was a couple years ahead of me. I was so grateful for the inside tips and strategies she provided that would help me in my job search.

I had been told repeatedly that obtaining a contract in the Ottawa board would take me at least five years. I did not speak French, and the system was flooded so there was a shortage of jobs. The list of hoops that one had to jump through was endless. Thankfully, I love a good challenge.

My first placement was in a little hamlet called Munster. It reminded me of home. I loved the small school, the huge schoolyard, and the sense of community in this public school. On day one I met my crew of other female teachers, and we connected right away. They were all heart and eager to learn new teaching practices. Once again I felt the comfort and support of a group of women.

I was a young teacher, full of energy and bright ideas. I was innovative and creative, and I wore my heart on my sleeve. The students gravitated to me like a magnetic force. Fully prepared, heart pumping and full of excitement, I walked into the classroom ready to teach my first lesson, one that looked at warm and cold colors with the inspiration of Kandinsky's abstract pieces and focus. The last student to introduce himself to me was Kyle, a student another teacher had "warned" me about. Apparently, he was a troublemaker and difficult to teach. I thanked her for her input but politely said that I didn't agree with labels. I was triggered, as it sent me straight back to the grade school experiences with labels that my brother and I had been given. I set out to change that and it would start that very day.

As I walked around the room, observing and chatting with the students about their technique and application of the lesson, I noticed that Kyle was painting his arms instead of the large sheet of paper. I smiled and headed in his direction. He stopped what he was doing, looked straight up at me, and fully prepared himself for the discipline he expected. Instead, I said, "Kyle, you can continue to paint your arms or even the desk. As long as you show me that you've gained the concept of warm/cold colors and the idea behind Kandinsky's abstract art, I will grade your art right here and now. I ask that you do not bother any of your neighbors, and that you clean up after yourself." At the end of our class period, Kyle earned an A. And he cleaned up his station and everyone else's, washed all the paintbrushes, and helped prepare for the next class. I "saw" him, and he knew it.

From that day on, Kyle started to shine. That sparked a surge in me, and I made it my mission to make sure that all my students experienced their own shining moment. I could and would teach anything, just to get them to see how amazing their minds were and how capable they could be. I wanted to create real-life magic for my students, show them the wonders of the world, and instill in them the "knowing" that someone believed in them. That was my recipe. That way, they would blossom. I ended my placement year with a number of schools asking me to return the following year as a supply teacher. Most exciting, however, was the offer of a part-time contract at Munster. I was well on my way and feeling unstoppable.

After celebrating our first year in Ottawa, Darryl and I decided it was finally time for just the two of us to find a place to live. We went shopping for dishes, kitchen utensils, and all the stuff. We made our first apartment a home in no time and had a great year together.

That summer, we booked a twenty-one-day backpacking trip to Europe. It was a trip of a lifetime. We based our plans around things that we loved to do: eat, drink wine, hike mountains, ride trains, and sit on beaches. The trip was beyond full of amazing moments, big and small, that we shared together.

One of those experiences was a hike up the Bernese Oberland Railway to the designated climb of Eiger Mountain, Switzerland. Darryl had wanted to take a detour to a lookout spot with the best view of Mount Jungfrau. Eager to arrive, I walked ahead, completely in awe of the most beautiful mountains I had ever seen. Meanwhile, Darryl spent the trek talking nonstop, saying things that in truth, I was not paying any attention to because I was too swept away by the scenery. Little did I know that he was professing his love and devotion to me. At one point I turned around to find him down on one knee, and before I could even clue into what he was doing, I told him to stand up to take a photo with me. He stopped me, took my hand, then pulled a tiny box out of his pocket. Inside was a princess-cut diamond on a gold band. My dream engagement ring. Nervously, he asked, "Ashley, will you marry me?" Switzerland became just the start of our adventures, the place I said yes, and the next big chapter.

That December I was told of an opening in a public school in Kanata. Without a second thought, I wrote up my application and sent it in. I knew that there would be hundreds of applicants, but I had to at least try. I understood then and still do that opportunities come and go, and that you'll miss every opportunity you don't go after.

I got an interview! That day, my walk and talk displayed every ounce of my confidence. I knew I was a fabulous teacher. I was full of heart, passion, and dedication. I knew I was going after this job with everything I had. The interview panel asked one final question: "Miss Ashley, is there anything else you would like to tell us about why we should hire you?" I did not flinch. I held strong and true. With a smile, I delivered the most honest and bold answer to date: "Yes, whether you hire me or the school down the road does, I will get a contract and flip any school for the better, for I am an amazing teacher." I shook their hands, thanked them for their time, and told them that I looked forward to hearing back from them soon.

And I did. I heard back immediately. I had gotten the position.

Once again, I was at a new school, which meant meeting new staff and all new students. The students responded to my energy, and right away, we connected. Trust was established and the excitement and eagerness to learn was palpable. These students were amazing.

One March morning, my principal was full of smiles upon my arrival. He had big news and just couldn't wait to share it. After years of dedication to working and pouring all my energy into my job and students, I finally heard the words "the contract is yours." That morning, I was handed a full-time teaching contract and acceptance into a leadership program. I was handed my dream. I was at the top of the ladder. I'd made it!

Bubbling over with excitement and with no time to tell Darryl my news, I took the girls' volleyball team to their tournament that was scheduled for that day. The team and I arrived ready to play and ready to win! The energy flowing through me was electric, and they could all feel it. We were supercharged. We won our first game but lost our second. Our overall points secured our spot in the semifinals. Before our game, we gathered together to eat lunch and wait to be called to play. Then my cell phone rang.

Darryl paused, waited for me to get outside, and then like a bomb, dropped the news that he was matched to London, Ontario, beginning on July 1. I stopped breathing. I couldn't speak. Tears poured from my eyes. Tiny snowflakes dropped on my nose as I sat in the parking lot with the news of our complete life change.

Darryl must have said my name a dozen times before I snapped out of it. "Yes, I heard you . . . we are moving to London." I knew that this would be the best career move for him. London was ranked number one, and that day, so was Darryl. I mustered up the strength to congratulate him and told him that I would see him at home. I held my news under my breath as I hung up the phone.

I've experienced panic attacks before. Many times in university, right before exams or a large paper, I would feel the tightness in my chest, the loss of breath, and the fear creep in. In each of these moments, I knew who to call and where to find him. My dad, my sounding board and voice of reason and comfort. He would know what to do and how to get me through it.

I can still hear his soothing voice telling me that it would all be okay. "Ashley, the world works in the most mysterious ways and things will unravel in time to show you why they occurred in the first place. Congratulations on getting your contract. Now stand up, take a big breath in, and get back to your team. They need a leader; now go be one." Softly I recentered, repeated my mantra "just breathe," and did just that. I went back to the girls.

To say that I had my brave face on when I delivered the news to my colleagues would be a lie. I was a puddle and could barely look them in the eye. Reality sunk in. We were set to move to London at the end of June. I declined the contract position just hours after I'd received it.

Saying goodbye to Ottawa was one of the hardest goodbyes I have ever made. I loved the city, and I had worked my ass off in those short four years. I had reached the top and celebrated every step along the way with nights out in the Byward Market with amazing girlfriends. It was my happy place. My home. It was also the place where six months earlier, Darryl and I had said I do.

The morning of my move, I hesitated to start the car. I knew that the second I started driving that the move to London would become my new reality—and it wasn't a reality I had picked for myself. I was supporting my husband's dream and the next steps in his career. What I was actually doing was showing up for him and not for my own dreams. It was a compromise, a heartbreaking one.

I wanted to be a principal, a great leader in a system that needed them. I wanted to change the world for the children who were not seen in an education system. Smart, capable children that were forgotten about or labeled "troublemakers," "slow," or "bad eggs." It was my mission to correct the system that failed my brother and me, a system that called us "stupid." I'd promised my brother and my younger self that I would be a powerful woman. It was my goal to be a role model for all the little girls who needed a warrior. To be that someone who would hear them, believe them, and stand so strong for them.

Yes, I just left my dream job and yes, I felt resentment toward my husband for making me leave it all behind me. But like with any new beginning, I was presented with a challenge that I could choose to embrace. I would take it on and seek out my new potential.

While I drove the distance, Darryl, already in London, had begun the process of setting up the furniture and putting the kitchen together. He knew that I was making this journey for him and was full of emotions. Smart man. I arrived, and we had little time to unpack. His orthopedic residency was to start shortly, and we decided that the unpacking would have to wait. We headed to my family's home to celebrate the Canada Day weekend.

It was wonderful to be with my family again. That weekend I sat poolside, my legs dangling in the water, chatting with Darryl and my mom. We were having fun and joking around about how my brother was at his best friend's house with all his buddies, most likely up to no good. My mom even made a joke that someone would come away with a broken neck.

What seemed like moments later, my brother's best friend called us with life-altering news: yes, someone had had an accident, and that someone was my brother, Justin. With the phone in one hand and my body moving at supersonic speed, I jumped into action mode with Darryl. We arrived at the scene before the ambulance. Darryl, a newly graduated doctor and an orthopedic resident, was the perfect person to be by Justin's side. Me, his sister, the warrior of the family, was the second best.

From day one of his life, I'd been Justin's big sister and his biggest defender. In one instance, I even peed on a park bench after a bunch of bullies were making fun of him because he had wet his pants—a condition that he could not control. So, I peed on the bench too and then laughed at this group of assholes for not being cool enough and powerful enough to control their own bladders enough to pee on demand. "Losers," I said.

On the day of Justin's accident, Darryl got him stable and assisted the paramedics while I took in all the surrounding details like a detective. Justin and his buddies had made a "slip and slide" that pointed down the hill and toward a large plastic pool. Repeatedly, the big university-aged men went down the slide and into the pool, earning the reward of a beer or some sort of booze at the end of the ride.

When we arrived at our small-town hospital, Justin was taken directly into the ER with Darryl accompanying him. I was greeted by my devastated parents and shocked sisters. As a family unit, we not so patiently waited for news. A while later, Darryl walked slowly out of the ER to deliver it to us.

Justin had a C5 and C4 burst fracture of his neck and would be airlifted to a hospital in Toronto within the hour. Darryl would be accompanying him in the helicopter, and we were asked to meet them there. We couldn't believe it. In disbelief, we headed to the car.

Hearing the words "he should be dead or a quadriplegic" out of the doctor's mouth had been enough to bring us all to our knees. The doctors had told us Justin's options were to have surgery to fuse his neck, a procedure that would immobilize him, or he could undergo the application of a halo to secure his neck in place until it healed. He made the decision to try the halo and start his healing journey that afternoon.

In Toronto, we gathered in Justin's hospital room. High on pain-killers, he lay on the bed with four holes drilled into his head holding the 30 lb halo that kept his neck stabilized. We held everything else. The lights were low, and for a moment, everything was calm. That didn't last long.

Without warning or any form of communication or preparedness, several nursing staff with a high sense of urgency entered the room, flicked on the overhead fluorescent lights, and yanked his hospital bed out into the hallway. They were in a mad rush to get him out of the room and inadvertently put him into full survival mode in the process. Justin's face went green and his eyes showed pure panic. I yelled at the top of my lungs, "STOP! STOP! He's going to throw up!"

Sure enough, Justin opened his mouth and vomit shot into the space above him and hit the ceiling before landing directly on his head, face, and new halo, which had a thick layer of sheep wool to protect his skin. He was covered in his own vomit and the nursing staff kept rushing his bed down the hallway. I ran behind them, shouting for them to stop. They reached his room and with full force, slammed the head of his bed against the wall. My dad, directly behind me, witnessed everything and fell to the floor in shock and stress.

Without a second to think, and in an eerier tone of voice than I have ever used with anyone, I slowly and calmly told the nursing staff to get the fuck out of the room. Justin's eyes filled with tears. His face was hot with pain and fear. I gently cleaned up the vomit the best I could and told him that I would handle the situation. "Trust me," I said. "I've got you." I stood in my fierceness and in my power and told my inner self to buck up. Justin was alive, and it was no time for me to cry. I had him to care for and protect.

Justin was two weeks post accident and was gaining more modality, strength, and confidence with his new halo on a daily basis. As for the family, we were all adjusting too. I had decided to take the rest of the summer off and stay with him. The unpacking in London could wait. I occupied my time with running, swimming, taking care of Justin, and/or keeping him company, as well as connecting with old friends. One of my best friends from university who'd moved out west after graduation was coming home to Ontario for her bachelorette party and wedding in August. The heartache from Justin's accident and our move from Ottawa had put a lot of stress on me, and it was time for me to unwind, let go, and have some fun.

The night of the bachelorette, my friends and I danced up a storm. Then, near the stage, I saw one of my friends yelling at a bouncer; her arms were definitely telling him right where to go, which led to all of us being ushered off the stage and out the door.

Somewhere in the commotion of it all, I lost my balance and went tumbling down a flight of stairs. Without thinking, I got up and then promptly fell again. My foot grew in size and the pain hit. My wing woman and dance partner for the night was the daughter of the city fire marshal, and she called for a pickup. Thirty minutes later, which was enough time to sober up and truly feel the throbbing of my injury, I got picked up by firefighters and the big truck! We departed in style and got dropped at my friend's house for the night.

The next morning, I had to make the call to my mom and arrange for her and my sister Sarah to come pick me up and drive my car home. When they arrived, my mom took one look at me and almost laughed. She knew she wasn't taking me home but straight to the hospital for an x-ray.

Back at the small-town hospital and ironically with the same doctor who treated Justin just weeks before, I heard the doctor tell my mom to put bubble wrap around us! As for my treatment, I would be on crutches with an air boot for at least four to six weeks.

The look on Justin's face when I slowly, with my head low, crutched into the living room was priceless. What was there to do but laugh at me and this ridiculous situation? The bubble wrap joke made sense to everyone, including me.

A couple weeks later, when I was fully functional and rather quick on my crutches, I decided it was time for me to return to

London, see my husband, set up our apartment, and look into getting a job. It was time to start my new life. It was time for my next transition.

HERstory

RACHEL

"My prime adult dating years felt like they were slipping through my fingertips. Processing the breakup, the COVID isolation, and the concept of adulthood, I fell into the trap of comparing my life to others and felt like I was getting left behind. I decided to do something completely out of my comfort zone, and that changed everything."

Fresh out of university, Rachel was ready to take on the adult world and make those forever connections: job, sense of self and adventures, house and home, and a partner with whom to enjoy it all. She quickly completed the first item on the adult checklist by landing a job that would take her to a new town. There, she met "the boy." He came into her life, swept her off her feet, and checked off all the boxes for what a perfect partner "should" be like.

Everything was falling into place and the next steps were planned out. "I was coming up on my one-year anniversary with my boyfriend and figured that before our two-year anniversary we would be engaged." It was all aligned, until it wasn't.

This boy pulled a complete stop with a simple question: "Are you happy with our relationship?" The answer changed everything, and Rachel, only one hour later, was devastated and alone. Her thoughts ran wild with questions: Had there been red flags?

Why had this happened so suddenly? Where had she gone wrong? Could she have changed something? She felt completely blindsided and was searching for answers. She hadn't realized that he was unhappy in their relationship, and it felt as though someone had taken her feet out from underneath her. According to her life plan, he was a man who would ask her to marry him and have children with her.

The thing about being blindsided by anything is that after the ground settles, the real lesson reveals itself. Rachel slowly began to process the layers of their relationship. In doing so, she realized how disconnected they had been. Her checklist that included finding the "perfect" partner combined with feelings of settling and pressures of being IN a relationship were totally opposite to what she actually wanted in life.

She sought help from friends and a therapist to come to terms with the realization that there had been a lot of red flags. What she thought and what was real were totally different. This growth did not come easy for Rachel. The layers she was uncovering connected to her own beliefs, self-talk, and a disconnect to her inner self, something that was harder for Rachel to deal with than the actual breakup itself. The breakup had simply been the catalyst for this discovery.

"I threw myself into work, joined a book club, signed up for a hockey team, visited out-of-town friends on weekends, and kept every spare moment as busy as possible. Although I was processing the breakup over time, I couldn't shake the question in my head: 'Well, now what?'"

Then March 2020 arrived and Rachel, like the rest of the world, entered the global pandemic. Feelings of comparison and lack overcame her while she sat alone scrolling through social media. She saw pictures and read stories about friends finding love and having children; their lives seemed to continue despite the lockdowns.

Rachel felt like her prime dating years were slipping through her fingertips. Although she had made headway since the breakup, she slipped back into a state of sadness. She missed her friends and companionship, and she was at a complete loss as to what she would do with her life going forward.

When she realized that there was no direction to go but up, Rachel stepped out of her comfort zone. She joined a learn-to-run series where she was introduced to other women who also had an interest in running. From there, she said yes to other activities and new adventures. She went from questioning what to do next to hiking new trails and having deep conversations and connections with inspiring women from all over. They became mentors to Rachel, and listening to their stories of heartache, successes, failures, great loves, and even motherhood, Rachel felt a sense of community.

Rachel soon experienced a newfound love for running, which opened her up to new challenges with distances. She went from running shorter distances to completing her first half marathon. She was blossoming; she was finding herself and confirming that there was so much more to life than her past checklist and breakup.

"Reflecting on the past three years, I would say it is true that time heals everything. I was devastated by the breakup, but I am so grateful that it happened. I would have never achieved personal growth without that experience. I know that I definitely don't have this adult life figured out, and I don't know what transition is next for me. But I am learning to be comfortable with the uncomfortable."

VANESSA

"Standing alone on the beach, white roses in hand and after running the most challenging race of my life, I said my goodbyes, accepted forgiveness, and released myself from carrying the heavy load of shame over my decision. I chose my life. My body, heart, and soul were coming home and healing, and I was committed to seeing my dreams come true."

Growing up as a child of Italian immigrants, Vanessa had heard all the stories of the hardships and tough times her family had experienced in the move to Canada after World War Two. Her parents had strived to provide more for their kids, and so Vanessa was privileged to experience an upper-middle-class lifestyle, while at the same time deeply knowing the emotion of fear that scarcity and financial hardship can cause. Vanessa felt the weight of the lessons her parents had instilled in her about the importance of being able to provide for herself financially and create a foundation of financial stability for her family.

These lessons remained with Vanessa as she grew into a young adult. She experienced a deep knowing that her heart's passions for playing music and cooking would not likely turn into her career if she wanted to become the independent woman who could take care of herself and create the financial future she desired. Vanessa entered her thirties on an upward climb to figure out what living her dreams looked like and how she would get there.

Shortly after her thirtieth birthday, Vanessa and her partner of two years found themselves honoring the life of his grandmother. They stood at her bedside, said their goodbyes, and held hands all the way home from the hospital. Vanessa, very intuitive, felt the energy shift and become supercharged with the need for love and comfort, for both her and him.

"I can remember the moment that the baby was conceived. It was a conversion of all the energies of that day. In the moments directly following our lovemaking, we got the phone call that his grandmother had just died. There was something about the timing of everything."

A few weeks later, after days of feeling unwell, Vanessa took a pregnancy test and discovered that she was indeed pregnant. It was not part of her plan at the time. Unsure what to do or how to respond to the news of her pregnancy, she did her best to hide the evidence from her work colleagues and family. When one of her coworkers caught on and approached her, Vanessa confided in her partner. He was still grieving and did not feel like he was financially secure enough on his own to provide for them or to take on the role of a father. Vanessa had finished law school a year earlier and was new to a small firm. She hadn't yet established herself as a practicing lawyer, and she had years of schooling expenses to pay off.

For weeks they discussed whether having the child was the right choice. Vanessa struggled. In her heart, she knew she wanted the baby. She had always wanted to be a mother, but she also took into consideration other factors: obligations, judgments and disappointment, financial stress, career aspirations, and the traditional roles of her culture.

Vanessa's health was also not ideal. She was still recovering from burnout and adrenal fatigue from years of law school. She was stressed, smoking, and not taking vitamins; simply put, she was not taking care of herself. Her body was already taxed, and now it was taken over by the symptoms of pregnancy, conflicting emotions, and complete overwhelm. Keeping her pregnancy a secret was painful and isolating. She knew that whatever they decided, she would be giving up a dream—a dream that included being a mother and raising her children with the security and resources to do the best job possible.

Vanessa and her partner ultimately decided that they were just not ready for a child; they were not ready to be parents.

On December 21, her partner drove Vanessa to the clinic, and when her name was called, he said goodbye to her before she entered the door. She had to do "the walk" by herself. The weight of the choice was on her heart, and her head hung low. Vanessa, heartbroken, cried.

When the procedure was over, Vanessa was taken to the recovery room where she was met with numerous other women who had also undergone the same procedure. Each woman had their own story, reason, situation, and circumstance. Each of them experienced deep loss and pain, emotionally, physically, and spiritually.

Vanessa hadn't told anyone, not even her own mother. She had no one to talk to, to confide or take comfort in. As the holiday festivities began, Vanessa felt more alone than ever. She was empty.

Isolated. Then the COVID lockdowns began, which heightened Vanessa's loneliness.

Transitioning to a legal career that was now being served remotely due to the pandemic, Vanessa had time to think about and reflect on what she had given up, both personally and professionally. She wasn't gaining ground in her career, nor was she getting any more traction toward financial security than she would have as a musician or a chef.

She had made huge sacrifices and given up on her creative dreams, and for what? She decided that she wanted to make an impact on the world. She had given up so much, including her opportunity to be a mom and have that baby, so she was going to make damn sure that she was going to put herself in a position to never have to make that decision again.

She had the tools, the education, the experience, and the ovaries to bring heart and soul to the world of law and the women who needed it. Vanessa would not be tied down to the suit. She created a new opportunity by breaking the box.

"I started to learn about entrepreneurship. I felt the surge of my soul's purpose. I felt empowered to become my own boss. I saw that being a lawyer was just part of the bigger picture. I had the tools to do it. I would help other people get there—they wouldn't have to give up their dreams for the feelings of security."

Vanessa's inspiration came from surrounding herself with a community where she witnessed other women who followed their hearts, created their businesses, and earned financial support in their own lives. She knew how to help people start businesses. If they could do it, so could she. The lesson imprinted, and with no plan, she quit her job and started out on her own.

Vanessa created new life goals and got to work on establishing her business. She also committed to improving her health and body. She knew that to achieve her business goals, she would have to have energy and stamina. Thus, she had to make her health a priority.

A friend of hers asked if she would join her in running an upcoming half marathon race in British Columbia. Vanessa jumped at the opportunity and started training. She joined a Girl Time Inc. run and yoga program, and with the support of that community, she did the work. Her time and energy were focused on following the program, doing the running, and taking in all the lessons and education on entrepreneurship in order to get her own law firm off the ground and running.

Vanessa flew out to BC alone and laced up for the most challenging race of her life. She got in the zone, ran the hills, and did not stop until she passed the finish line in tears. This moment was so much more than completing a race. She took back her power, gained confidence in herself, and did the soul work to get her to a place where she could open her heart to believe in herself. Forgiveness came next.

Post race, and after taking time to celebrate her victory, she bought a bouquet of white roses at a local store. In a meditative state, she slowly walked the path along a hiking trail by the Pacific Ocean, reflecting on the journey and the outcome of it all. It was a sad yet liberating moment for Vanessa, one that changed something deep inside of her: she shifted from a heavy energy full of shame to the lightness of being proud of what she had created.

It was here that her footsteps took her to the water's edge where a wash of emotion and a flood of tears came to the surface. She finally understood that the idealistic pursuit of financial security had cost her far too much: her dreams of being a musician, and then a chef, and the most heartbreaking, a child that would have been her own. She surrendered to the lesson, forgave herself, then allowed the water to wash it all away as she threw the roses into the ocean.

For Vanessa, the greatest life lesson came in her thirty-third year and with the heart-opening realization that all her decisions had led to that moment by the ocean. Any decision, journey, adventure, challenge, climb, and transition that came next in her life would be met with heart, soul, and purpose, and she was ready for it all.

YOURstory

Transitions are inevitable in life. Along with transitions come choices. Some are easy, but some are life changing and possibly, heartbreaking. But no matter what kind of choice one makes, it almost always comes with a lesson. Lean into that lesson and learn from it. You just may realize that you needed it to move forward in the right direction.

REFLECTION:

What choices have you made that have created the biggest lessons in your life? Have you ever had to give something up, only to find that you've gained something in return?

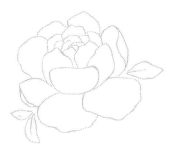

Chapter 7: Motherhood

It was time for me to return to work, but I was at a loss. I'd been a contract teacher and leader in Ottawa, but my contract did not carry over to London and I knew absolutely no one. I would have to start at the beginning, at the bottom of the ladder, and jump all the hoops once more—a process that had taken me years and a ton of energy in Ottawa.

I was less than keen to start again and felt deflated from the summer lows and injuries. To me, the only option was to go back into retail; I'd have to get a sales job. At least there I could meet some people and earn some money until I felt the energy, motivation, desire, and ambition to start climbing the teaching ladder once again.

Still on crutches, I hobbled into an interview at one of the stores in the mall. A manager, who was leading the group interview, went straight in with a question about my injury. So I asked her, "Do you want the I-want-the-job version? Or do you want the truth about what really happened?" She nodded to the second option. The next thing I knew, I was hired. Who knows what they thought, but that day when I got home from my interview, I had a job and had made one hell of an impression on my new management team.

Darryl had started branching out as well. Under the ortho umbrella of residents, the senior class was hosting socials to bring some balance to the rigidity of the program and so people could introduce themselves and their partners. I met my first friend in London at one such social. This friendship brought some relief to the loneliness I was experiencing due to being new to the city. I was also soon making friends at work and the gym, and my joy began to return.

About a month into my new job, Justin called to inform me that his halo was being removed early and asked if I would meet him and our parents in Toronto. I didn't hesitate. I was thrilled to join my family to celebrate Justin's recovery, and it just so happened to also be my twenty-seventh birthday!

After that experience—seeing my brother walk without his halo and all the emotions it evoked for my family—I felt a significant nudge. Why wait? Life was happening around us. So, to Darryl, I said aloud a dream I had since I was a little girl playing dolls and Barbies: "Let's have a baby." Darryl and I giggled as we ran to the bedroom in hopes of starting a new chapter in our lives.

I realized that my dream had come true one day in a hot yoga class when I nearly fainted. My friend looked at me, laughed, and said, "Oh, girl, you look like shit. Go home and sleep it off." Well, I went home and instead of sleeping it off, I took a pregnancy test. There it was, the little blue plus symbol. I wasn't sick. I was pregnant.

As my belly grew, so did my anticipation of what motherhood would bring. Darryl and I began house hunting, and we bought all the baby gear and necessities. This new adventure in adulthood was full of change and making lifelong dreams come true. After signing the papers on our very first house together, I laughed over the realization that I was living out the pretend life of my Barbie: I'd gone off to school, gotten married, bought a house and now, I was about to push a baby in a baby carriage.

It was 4 a.m., and I woke up in panic thinking that I peed our bed. Darryl decided that we should go to the hospital to make sure that the baby and I weren't experiencing any stress. I didn't put much thought into it; I was thirty-six weeks pregnant, it was too early to be thinking about delivery. I threw on some clothes, grabbed my purse, and walked out the door. I was super tired, and I knew I had to work in the morning.

We were greeted by one of the intake nurses who listened to why we had come into the hospital. She passed us the paperwork to fill out and said with a laugh, "Um, girl, you're not leaving this hospital without a baby. You are in labor." She was right. A couple hours later, Lillian was born. The second she screamed, I, too, was born. My name changed, my world expanded, I spoke a new language, and I was initiated into the "mom club." I suddenly had totally different priorities, needs, and wants. My heart had never known such love. It had never known this level of fear, protectiveness, and fierceness. It truly was the biggest change in the shortest period of time. One minute I'd been pushing, and the next, I became a mom.

Leaving the hospital and bringing a newborn baby home is surreal. There's no manual and no real preparation. You rely on your support team, your intuition, and your gut feelings, plus the hope that you are going to learn by doing. It's the trial-and-error approach. I hadn't read the books, and I didn't belong to a mommy group. So there I was, a new mom in my new house; it was just Lillian and me.

Darryl was a second year ortho resident. He was working an insane number of hours and was always on call. At any moment, he'd jump up and leave without warning. I rarely saw him. He would return home after his shift, and I'd already be in bed after a whole day of changing diapers, washing laundry, and figuring out how to keep Lillian (and myself) alive. Our worlds did not match up. When he was home, he was sleeping so as to regain his energy to return to the hospital.

Loneliness and resentment were inching their ugly selves into our sleep-deprived lives, and our degree of separation grew wider. We had zero time together for even the little things—the moments that I fully expected and dreamed of having before Lillian was born. You know, movie moments like when you see new parents watching their baby sleep in awe and amazement over what they created together. Darryl and I had no such moments.

Lillian was only a couple weeks old when I noticed that her breathing was labored and she was coughing up mucus after every feeding. Thankfully, Lillian was a natural latcher, and my breast milk came in without any worries. But the worries that came post feeding were intense. Lillian would scream bloody murder, arch her back, then vomit all the milk plus mucus. Mix that with the lack of sleep and I was a complete hot mess the first eight weeks into motherhood. A successful day for me was one when I remembered to brush my teeth. It was worth celebrating. I didn't know many women who had a baby before I did, so I only had vague stories from my mom and mother-in-law to lean on, which didn't provide much comfort those early weeks.

Slowly but surely, Lillian and I got into our own little routine. When she would sleep, I would clean up, do prep work, or sit in our quiet living room reading and dreaming of being social again. Many times, I'd daydream of being a part of a mommy group or having other mommy friends with whom I could walk and attend playdates. I saw little groupings of mothers strolling in the neighborhood or when I walked the mall on rainy days, and I felt envy over their companionship. I desperately wanted a community, a group to belong to.

Jayne (Justin's girlfriend) and my friend Laura were having a party, and I decided to take Lillian with me. I was desperate for some girl time. Although I received a warm welcome, I was out of place. My friends were excited to see Lillian, to hold her and ask how I was doing, but when she would cry, was hungry, or needed her bum changed, it was a different story. My friends were focused on getting ready for a night out, laughing and sharing party or guy stories, and I was focused on surviving the night without breaking down crying. So I thanked Jayne and Laura for inviting me, and I made my exit.

After that night, I questioned how I was going to find and make friends now that I was home with a baby, had no support or babysitter, and was still relatively new to the area. This new world was so beyond foreign to me. I felt like an alien, estranged from normal civilization. Before having Lillian, I'd thought I was lonely in London. Now, after having Lillian, I was lonely and a mother.

I soon realized that my challenge over finding my place, whether it was London, at home with family, or anywhere in the world, first started with my ability to find myself within my new identity. I was not the same Ashley, as I'd changed the very second Lillian was born. I was Lillian's mother, and Lillian was my guide. She knew my rhythm and flow, and she responded first to them. My job was to figure everything out and learn from our experiences.

Our first winter together, I would be reminded of this lesson multiple times and in multiple ways. Lillian was all of six months old when I came down with the flu. I was ridiculously sick. I had a fever and zero energy to lift my head. I made Lillian a little bed on the bathroom floor out of towels and her baby blanket and then lay beside her on the cool tiles.

Darryl was at the hospital, and in desperation, I called my mom. I needed help. I needed my mom. My tears dropped as my mom told me that no, she wouldn't be making the long drive and that I could handle it myself. I acknowledged her response and said I understood. It was winter, the roads were icy, and she had animals to look after. Still, my heart broke. I nodded my head. I understood what I needed to do and who was going to do it for me.

It is truly amazing how resilient and adjustable one can be when they are pushed to their limit. In my first year of being a mom, I was pushed so far past my comfort zone, so far past my limit and what I thought I was capable of, that I found myself embracing change in any and every way possible. I knew I had to relearn who I was: as a mother, yes, but also as a friend, a partner and wife, and a daughter. What felt like a heartbeat ago, I'd been teaching, coaching volleyball and running, and excelling as a leader in my school; then I was a warrior for my brother and was the reserved new girl at my sales job. Now I had a baby and was changing diapers, cleaning house, teaching her sign language, and playing with blocks and squeaky toys. I desperately wanted alone time to work out or read a book, and I desperately wanted to be a part of a community. In the shortest period of time, I'd completely changed my life, and in truth, I could barely recognize the woman I'd once been. Time flies, and not just when you are having fun.

As my twenty-ninth birthday approached, the need to find myself again became more apparent to me. It was constantly on my mind. I questioned how I could bring back the "old" Ashley and introduce her to "new" Ashley's world. I wanted to somehow combine these worlds and find my spark again. I missed it, and I knew that the only one to reignite that spark was me. I was ready to blossom yet again.

The last time I'd done any goal setting or mapped out any activity, personal growth, or self-love and dedication was when I attended a leadership conference in Toronto. While in a boardroom with other future leaders, we did a goal-setting exercise that was referred to as "Blue Sky: Living Your BEST life." Essentially, "blue skies" meant that anything and everything was possible. The sky isn't even the limit.

The task asked us to visualize living our best life, every detail. We'd then write it out in the present tense as though we were already living it. Next, we'd create all the action steps that would get us from our words to action and toward making those "blue sky" visions a reality. I absolutely LOVED the workshop. It completely engaged me and I wrote out every detail of what the future Ashley's life looked like.

As a new mom, I realized something was missing. It was "I" who was missing. My baby was happy and I was in love with her little toes, sweet little laughter, and how much fun it was to make her smile, but my marriage was disconnected, my friendships were distant, my body was longing for energy, and my soul was aching for its spark to return. I was not aligned with *me*. It was time for me to reconnect to myself and my "blue sky" life.

I proceeded to make a list of thirty things I was going to do before I turned thirty. I had always loved a good challenge, so I took the time to really think about what I wanted in my life. I wrote down all the activities I loved doing, then took it one step further and created a vision board. I cut out images of items from my list, including a little piece of paper that said, in handwriting, "Baby boy, January/February." I made sure to place my list and my vision board in a spot where I would see them daily. They were to be my reminders to bring Ashley back to life.

HERstory

SHANNON

"It wasn't supposed to be like this. You are supposed to fall in love the second you hold your newborn, and all I wanted to do was drift off into the silence of the dark water of Georgian Bay."

Shannon was beyond excited to find out she was pregnant. She had known the pain of losing a child after experiencing a miscarriage in her previous relationship, and she was ready to open her heart to a new relationship, a new life, and the opportunity to become a mom, a new role for her.

Shannon and her partner, Colin, had *everything* planned out and prepared. A high-caliber woman, Shannon always committed one hundred percent to everything she did. She and Colin wanted to enter their life together as a growing family feeling ready. Although feelings of anxiety and fear surfaced while carrying her baby, Shannon met them with excitement and pride that her body was healthy—she was a lifelong athlete naturally gifted in sports—and she was able to reach full term in this pregnancy.

A natural delivery turned into a traumatic experience for Shannon when her baby got stuck in her birth canal. Her midwives had been concerned about the large size of the baby, and it took all of Shannon's strength to push out her ten-plus pound baby. Immediately, there was chaos among the midwives and the supporting nurses and doctor. Everyone began moving quickly. Shannon, meanwhile, started hemorrhaging. Her nerves were shot and her body went into stress mode due to blood loss. Her mental and physical fatigue and overwhelm imprinted trauma on her system and memory as a result. As for her baby, she was "whisked away," screaming the whole time.

The midwives returned with her newborn, all swaddled in a soft pink blanket and bonnet, and shocking news. Shannon and Colin's baby had been born with developmental dysplasia of the hips and would have to be fitted with a Pavlik Harness. Although Shannon worked in health care as a kinesiologist and has a master's degree in rehabilitation science, she was not able to fully process the information. Holding her newborn, who had not yet stopped screaming, Shannon had an unnerving feeling that everything was strange. She was stressed, confused, and traumatized—all feelings that made her think she had failed herself.

The first five days of their newborn's life were tumultuous. After the Pavlik Harness fitting was complete, a bilirubin blanket was also wrapped around the baby in order to treat neonatal jaundice. The screams continued, as the colicky newborn was unable to relieve gas pains due to restrictions of the harness and blanket. Under this amount of stress, Shannon's milk didn't fully come in, and with her baby in such discomfort and the harness making it very difficult to nurse, breastfeeding was not the bonding experience Shannon had hoped for. Additionally, they had been traveling back and forth to the hospital with zero rest or breaks. Shannon felt as if she couldn't function, and all she could hear were the constant screams of her baby, even when the baby was asleep or quiet. Shannon was haunted by the screams, and that broke her spirit. She was on edge.

Colin returned to work after two weeks, and Shannon became overcome with feelings of anger, resentment, frustration, comparison, and anxiousness. She questioned what she was doing "wrong" and why no one else seemed to be experiencing this or talking about it. Other mothers weren't sharing their dark stories. She felt entirely alone.

Although she tapped into the resources that her family doctor, the midwives, and family and friends suggested, she still couldn't see the light at the end of the tunnel of a screaming baby. Her baby's screams were like nails on a chalkboard. They reached the darkest parts of her, and there was no relief in sight.

"I couldn't breathe. I was suffering in silence and didn't understand why. Across our road is an entrance to the Bay. When Colin was home or someone was with the baby, I would walk there by myself and walk right into the water. I wanted the water to take me away. The waves calmed the screaming in my mind and settled my broken nerves. In the Bay, it was quiet."

It wasn't until one of her midwives connected her to another mom, a woman who had spoken up and experienced similar feelings to Shannon, that she got some relief. This was Shannon's introduction to a quiet community of other mothers. Finally, there were women who wanted to talk and share experiences, and that resonated with how Shannon was feeling, dealing, and coping with the weight of postpartum depression.

Shannon made the shift to reclaim her life. She started with self-compassion, sleep strategies, and schedules. She then continued with better eating, meal preparation, daily activity and physical outlets, and meditation and mindset activities. She took back her power by acknowledging what she needed as a woman, as a new mom with a baby who needed her to be her best.

Shannon's baby needed a healthy mom, and her knowing that made all the difference. Shannon had once been asked in an entrepreneurial meeting with other boss women what animal best represented her. Shannon chose a horse, describing herself as strong, loyal, determined, and fast. Shannon finally found herself again—she returned to being strong, loyal, and determined, just like a horse.

LINDSAY

"The journey into motherhood is not the same for everyone. My partner watched me transform into someone he didn't recognize, which left him without his best friend. For me, though, it was my journey to take."

Growing up, one of Lindsay's many strengths was in academics. Reading book after book, reaching for straight As, and striving for excellence is what fueled her and admittedly, still does. Her mother's fears of living life kept Lindsay on the sidelines, watching but never joining in and in a constant state of anxiety. Her comfort zone was the world of academia. That A+ in life was what she needed, and it is what she got.

When Lindsay met Blair, he broke her glass of perfection and brought with him a world of ease, which gave Lindsay the nudge to explore another side of herself. Blair brought out her playful side, a beautiful balance to a world of studying. First comes love, then comes marriage, then comes Lindsay pregnant and reading every book on pregnancy, babies, and parenthood.

Although reading book after book gave Lindsay the security that she was prepared, it also gave her more ideas and theories to contemplate and fixate on. Pregnancy is one full-body takeover, but birth? Birth is a completely different experience for every woman who has experienced it. Lindsay knew that no matter how many books she read, she would not know what would overtake her body and her body's need to take care of a little human.

All the books were read, the baby room was set up, the hospital bag was packed and ready; there was even time to inform the nurses just how "prepared" Lindsay was to have her first baby. Every detail had been planned out until it was time to push. Then things changed. Lindsay's delivery dramatically turned from a vaginal delivery to a C-section, and her nervous system regulation felt attacked.

"I pushed and pushed, and she didn't want to come. Then they sliced her out of me. My body felt like it was under an attack, which was a traumatic event for me, and I responded negatively to her, to my husband, to it all. I never expected this to happen. We never thought about or planned on a C-section."

Baby girl Quinne was born and Lindsay, a new mom whose nervous system was unable to regulate itself, was born too. One topic in particular that had held Lindsay's attention during her pregnancy was postpartum obsessive-compulsive disorder. And now she was experiencing it.

According to Postpartum Support International, it is a disorder that can present itself during pregnancy and/or postpartum. New mothers experience a repetition of thoughts, worries, and actions about their child. Mothers repeatedly look to see if they are still breathing, as well as have recurring patterns of washing and rewashing bottles, baby toys, or clothing to cleanse them of germs and dirt. Additionally, they may obsessively check the baby monitor and practice other obsessive behavior.

For Lindsay, having a baby not only brought to the surface her OCD behaviors, but it also heightened her awareness about her childhood triggers, fears, and need for healing. Lindsay's need to control everything took its toll on her, and she began projecting it onto Quinne.

Unable to fully comprehend the severity of Lindsay's surgery and the extent of her recovery from the C-section plus her feelings of being "wrecked," Blair felt blocked. Their once-linked connection, best friend status, and partners-in-crime attitude was replaced by one of strangers. Blair could not do anything "right," and he was not in tune with what Quinne or Lindsay needed.

"He's a natural 'fixer' and does not do well when he feels useless. At that time, I simply didn't care what he needed. I felt like I was on my own. I had this crazy need to protect Quinne; not even my mom or mother-in-law were allowed to comfort her. I disconnected from Blair and grew resentful of the fact that he didn't have the capabilities to do what she needed—I was the only one who could."

A baby feels and responds to the emotions of the mother. In Lindsay's case, it wasn't until she noticed that Quinne was growing into her own personality and was beginning to show Lindsay what she wanted that the world wasn't as scary to her.

This realization plus the gentle reminder from her best friend and husband that there is no first place for the most worried mother—that her daughter would grow, develop, and show the world her own awesomeness, just as Lindsay had—did much to alleviate her fears.

The role of the parent is to nurture the individual spark that each child has, act as a guide throughout their life, and be a witness to their self-discoveries. Lindsay saw the opportunity to step back from the bridge she'd created and recognized the gravity that fear has on people. As a result, a shift happened (and almost overnight). The idea of continuing the cycle of trauma and imprinting it on

Quinne plus the disconnection she felt with Blair was enough to propel Lindsay into a new direction of motherhood and of self.

She implemented a daily gratitude practice and committed to regular exercise and meditation. Date nights with Blair were put on the calendar. Then together they introduced play, and not just for Quinne but alongside her too. She said, "I now do things to show Quinne independence. I got a road bike. I go running and practice yoga. I jumped off the pier. Even when Quinne wants me to stay home and 'stay safe,' I show her how to prioritize my health and well-being by going out." Little changes were big changes, and they all sparked joy.

Gradually, Lindsay dismantled the heavy guards of self-induced "perfections" and allowed a renewed sense of play, joy, and ease into her role as a mother and as a partner. The tiny fragile jar she'd been living in opened, and together with Blair, Lindsay found her new rhythm of parenthood.

"It has taken me years to find my joy, to try and enjoy parenthood. Children grow every day. Within the momentum of life, stop and enjoy the little things that they do. It makes it all so lovely. Don't be rushed—they notice you noticing the little things, and that's important. Make it fun!"

YOURstory

Motherhood does not come with a manual, and it is certainly not the same journey for everyone. The second her baby is born, a woman gains a new identity. She, too, is born; she has become a "mom." The adjustment can be difficult. She has a whole new world to discover about herself and her self-worth, and it can be an isolating and lonely experience. Finding a supportive community can be vital to a mother's journey and overall well-being.

REFLECTION:

In honoring our own definition of mom, we can honor ourselves. What does the word *mom* mean to you? What expectations do/did you attach to this word? Have you had the benefit of belonging to a community of women? If not, who can you rely on for support?

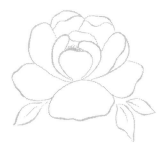

Chapter 8:
Relationship Challenges and Finding Grit

Darryl and I were living two different lives. Although our vision for our future together remained intact, our focus was not on each other. Quality time as a couple was not a priority. To the outside world, everyone believed it was because he worked such long hours in residency and I was focused on Lillian; to them, it was simply a "phase" we were going through. They had no idea the extent of our struggles; they had no idea the storm we were enduring.

Leaving Ottawa, declining my contract and dream job, saying goodbye to friends who were like family, and parenting alone most of the time had all taken a toll on me. London was proving to be more isolating and lonelier than I had expected. These layers of weight were damaging to my relationship, and resentment soon made a home in my heart where Darryl once lived.

Meanwhile, Darryl was just trying to survive. He was drowning in the heaviness of the residency program and the social expectations of and judgments about who he was expected to become. He had been placed on a pillar—a position that he did not want to be in and inadvertently, was out to destroy. All his time, energy, and effort were sucked up with his level of dedication to his job, a job that saved lives but was taking his.

Our London friends who were all under the umbrella of the ortho world understood the dedication it takes to complete residency and the sacrifices it requires from couples and families to endure it. These friends were our go-to people when we needed support or a safe place to confide. But even with them in place, Darryl and I could not reach each other, and slowly but surely, we drifted so far apart that by Valentine's Day, we found ourselves at our darkest time. Our relationship had hit rock bottom.

The severity of our situation came two weeks after Valentine's Day. I knew what being alone felt like and how it was changing me. I had just gotten myself back on my feet and was not about to take the fall with Darryl. So I packed suitcases for both Lillian and me and called Justin and Jayne to pick us up. I needed to go home to my family for help. When they arrived, their eyes were red with tears dropping. Jayne reached for Lillian and Justin for me. In my brother's arms, I released what was left of my energy and buried my head. I knew he could hold me up; I counted on it.

My parents were on vacation, which gave Lillian and me a few days at their home to adjust. I had no idea how long our stay would be. Justin and Jayne showed us love, compassion, support, and shelter from our self-made storm. There was no judgment, only love. I was so grateful.

My parents returned, and upon seeing the suitcases, my mom nodded her head and went to bed. My dad made our special drink—two glasses of rye and ginger with a splash of lime—and took a seat. He was my shoulder to cry on. We talked for hours. He spoke to me on a level that was not father to daughter but more like soul to soul. Before saying goodnight, my dad stood tall and proud in full faith that our fate as a couple was stronger than the ditch we had found ourselves in. Time, space, love, and compassion would bring healing.

Spring arrived and it was time for Darryl, Lillian, and me to be reunited. Lillian and I headed back to London where Darryl was waiting. We'd made the decision to seek therapy, and it began as we returned. Darryl and I slowly started to make our relationship a priority. We had date nights, long conversations, and time together as a family unit. Simple things like having our coffee together, walks, and park dates with Lillian were huge. Our therapy sessions gave us direction and tools for reuniting and acted as a safe space for us to dive deeper into ourselves and our marriage in order to find resolutions. It took effort, but it was all worth it. We were worth it.

Our marriage hadn't needed a final straw to break us. We needed a match. We needed to burn our marriage down to ashes so we could transform into a new life together with better versions of ourselves. We both needed to realize that it was not just one thing causing our division, but the whole picture. It was a true metamorphosis for our life as a couple, one where we experienced the death of our marriage and then the rebirth of it through joint attention, intention, focus, and vision.

We opened ourselves up in our conversations as if we were dating again. This time around, however, we skipped the honeymoon phase and dove straight into the importance of communication, connection, and trust. We knew not to rush the process but to let it flow naturally. We wanted to make sure we were both healing from our war wounds. Before we hit our bottom, we had discussed the possibility of having another baby. Now we needed to make sure we were aligned and connected enough to move forward as a couple.

We gradually became social again together. We went on adventures with other families and got out more in general. As Darryl and I rekindled our romance, I began feeling stronger physically, mentally, emotionally, and soulfully. I was running, practicing yoga, socializing, reading a ton of books, and dreaming of another amazing change. I was ready for another baby.

It had taken me one month to get pregnant with Lillian. Now, still in marriage recovery and knee-deep in residency, we had months of trying without a positive test. We did not start to really question our fertility until an unsettling conversation with close female family members sparked concern. From one, it was "What's wrong with you? When I wanted to become pregnant, it just happened, all four times." Another person's comment hurt the most: "Ashley, just because you can't get pregnant doesn't mean you have to take it out on us. We got pregnant right away; it's not our fault that you can't."

Pregnancy test after pregnancy test, the little blue line did not show up, but our worries, insecurities, inner pressures, and disappointment sure did. All combined, I started questioning whether there was something wrong with me. I have never been a patient person and trying to conceive the second time around proved to push my impatience to a whole new level. To make things more challenging, I didn't feel as if I had anyone to talk to about it. Infertility seemed to be a topic that was kept quiet.

After trying for six months without getting pregnant, Darryl and I decided that we should seek professional help and have some testing done. Our first appointment was a standard procedural one. We met with the specialist, and he asked us questions about our lifestyle, relationship, health, and careers. Basically, we walked him through our lives.

As soon as Darryl mentioned where he worked and what residency he was in, the doctor laughed out loud. He told us, in no uncertain words, that we would not get pregnant until we released control, relaxed, fully connected, and backed off the stressors in our lives. When we returned to his office a couple weeks later to get our test results, he let us know that while I was healthy, Darryl's body was under attack—it was exhausted and stressed. His whole body was reacting to the years of poor sleep, food, and nutrients. It was no wonder we were struggling to conceive: Darryl's body was weighed down by stress and was in survival mode, not reproduction mode.

With Darryl's upcoming rotations coming soon, we created a plan for how he was going to get his health back on track and how I was going to help him. We were in a good place in our marriage, and we were feeling confident in our future.

At the end of May, I had planned to take my first solo trip to Ottawa for a big race weekend. Lillian would spend the weekend with her grandparents, and I was looking forward to returning to the city I loved and to my best friends, Devon and Crystal. The focus was me and quality girl time. A weekend with friends was the magic I was looking for: running the race, going on dinner dates, getting dressed up, and dancing . . . a ton of dancing. My energy was on fire. That weekend refueled me. It breathed life back into every cell in my body.

Upon returning home to London with my "cup" overflowing with love from the weekend and then seeing Darryl after time apart, I completely forgot about trying for a baby. We were so excited to see each other.

Several weeks later, while back in London with my lifelong friend Shannon for a Dragon boat competition, I noticed that my energy was low and that things felt off. At the time I just figured it was due to my upcoming cycle, the constant changes, and traveling. I was wrong. Shannon knew the struggles we were having with conceiving and the distance Darryl and I had felt while we were away. She suggested a trip to the store. In the bathroom at Target, I took the test as Shannon held my hand. It did not take long for the double line to appear.

After a year of trying, I was pregnant, and just before Father's Day. Darryl got the best gift that year: a baby outfit and the pregnancy test that confirmed that patience and a focus on health and happiness and simply being together had worked.

As my tummy grew and my body changed, all the highs and lows of pregnancy took over. This time around, I had a toddler running around plus severe restless leg syndrome. I also tested positive for gestational diabetes. Considering my health, size, and lifestyle, this was rare. Regardless, I had it and this pregnancy was more challenging for me than my first.

Right around the twenty-week mark, we found out that we were having a baby boy. We also found out that all Darryl's efforts in his interviews for a fellowship had paid off. He was accepted into a number of fellowships all over Canada, and in the end, we decided that he would commit to one year in Toronto and one year in Banff, Alberta.

As the list of things to do to get ready for baby number two grew in length, so did the list of things to do to prepare our house for sale and get our move organized. Time was flying, and I was becoming overwhelmed with everything that had to be done. I really had to stay focused and in the zone to keep from spiraling. I had to find my grit.

By the time I was thirty-six weeks along, we made sure that our bag was packed and everything was arranged for Lillian's care. Sure enough, I went into labor early once again. At my next appointment, my doctor very calmly told me that I was 5 cm dilated. She told me to leave the office, call in my support team, get Darryl out of the OR, and grab my bag. Her voice, although calm, had a sense of urgency. She said that she would be seeing me again, and very soon.

The last time I'd heard that, I'd had a baby within a couple hours. So, I followed the doctor's orders, called Darryl, and made arrangements for Dawn, our family friend and huge supporter, to care for Lillian. Dawn was our family while living in London, and at that time, our only person to call.

At the hospital, we were thrown off with the rush of everything. Although my contractions were appearing on the screens, my body and my baby were not ready for full labor and delivery. We were told to walk, then walk some more. Patience is one virtue that I struggle with; when all I wanted to do was "go," being told to go slow and wait was a test for me. As it's said, "the struggle was real."

After a day and into the early night of walking, eating my third grape popsicle, and calling all my girlfriends, my body's ease changed directly into one of speed. My contractions hit me with fury; I went from a true zero to hero pain level. The nurses measured me, and the room changed. That is when Darryl said, "Hold!" He was not delivering our baby; I needed to wait for the doctor. I went inward, listened deep within my body, and found my strength to do just that: hold! The doctor arrived at 6:05 p.m. and our son, Everett, was born at 6:11 p.m. The wait was over. Our baby boy, born in February, had arrived. There he was, my Mount Everest, in my arms with a full head of black hair. My world had blossomed again. I was complete.

HERstory

ANNETTE

"Belonging starts from within. I knew I was different, right when I was put into my role of being female. I wanted to rebel, to go against all the rules and guidelines of the church, my parents, and the community. I knew judgment; I knew how everything worked and how everything was 'swept under the rug.' But I have a voice, hope, and the inner knowing that I am me—I am my own individual person. I fit with me, and I am woken."

In the midst of every hurricane, there is a break, a clearing when the sky opens up to reveal the blue behind the clouds. This clearing is the eye of the storm, the calm center of every tumultuous time or event. We know this pause. Some look at it as a sign that a storm, like all things, has a beginning and an end.

Adopted six weeks after she was born, Annette grew up in a Dutch reformed religious community. By nurture, she only knew her family's values, beliefs, and religious practices. By nature, though, she knew that she sat at a table where she didn't belong.

Fearful of outside influences, Annette's parents governed her experiences, right down to the simplest form of influence: television. Going against her family's rules, Annette sneaked in viewing time to watch *Beverly Hills, 90210*. The show fascinated her. In it, she saw women who spoke up. These characters had voices, and they used them. For Annette, watching these women on TV felt empowering, and she became curious about life outside her community.

At fifteen, Annette was well versed in what was expected of young girls and women, according to her family and the church: they were only to speak when spoken to; they were second-class citizens; they had to follow the laws of the church, house, and home; and acceptance was for followers, not outsiders. Although she was "popular" with the other kids in her community, Annette struggled with feeling as if she belonged, and she had numerous issues with the lack of rights and freedoms for women. She had feminist views, and that made her feel estranged.

"Women as leaders in the church? All hell would break loose. There were no women in leadership; none. As a female, you were only allowed to be a member of the choir. I angered my father whenever I brought up women in any sort of power. How dare I speak my mind? He always told me to be quiet, that the Bible had no errors and that a woman's place is in the home."

At eighteen, Annette became free to make her own decisions. It was as if the door of a birdcage had been opened. Annette met a young man who introduced her to drinking, smoking, speaking her mind, and seeking out opportunities to be seen as an equal. She was finally heard; her voice was welcomed. But freedom came at a cost. Their relationship was not meant for forever, and Annette was left with a growing baby inside her. She had only one option: to have the baby on her own.

Annette fully understood that she was soon to be a single parent and that meant big responsibilities and a total life adjustment. But having this baby also meant she would have someone in her life with the same bloodline. Thus, the baby became her world. Holding this love near and dear to her heart, she went home to inform her parents about the pregnancy.

"I was terrified to tell my parents. Sex before marriage was considered a huge sin. I thought my dad would become physical. Instead, he said, 'I hear you have a little problem. Don't worry, we will take care of you. Who is the father?' I was smart and quickly told him that it was a Catholic boy because I knew that would get me out of a wedding. And it did. I saw my out and took it."

Life did change dramatically for Annette. Even though her parents had strong opinions and beliefs, they showed up for her. They created a room in their home for Annette and the baby where they set up the crib and painted the walls pink. Baby girl Kianna was born, a true gift from above.

No stranger to the solo walk of shame, Annette stood in front of the church and publicly repented her sin. In doing so, she was welcomed back with open arms and into the household of a respectable young suitor: the church's golden boy and hero! While their dating was joyful, once Annette had his ring on her finger, their relationship changed and the rules, regulations, and roles returned to that of a "traditional" marriage in the eyes of the church.

Annette wanted more in life and struggled with this arrangement, one that expected her to stay home and have babies. She wanted education, and that included law school. She discussed her desire to attend law school with her new husband and his family, but she was shut down, something that shocked her. Her husband had supported the plan while they were dating, which was one of the reasons why she'd married him. Annette persisted, and her marriage ended a year and a half later despite the fact she was pregnant with her second child.

Annette, still standing firm in her decision to attend law school, had no choice but to figure out her next steps. Educating herself was the start. She got into school, committed to her studies and growth, and parented her two children. By twenty-nine, she owned her house, was a practicing lawyer, and was back in the dating world. Little did she know that she was in the eye of the storm.

Enter husband number two! Annette, still part of her family and church community, felt the pressure and fear of excommunication for being a single mother of two. As a result, she entered into another marriage after only seven months of dating. Her daughter, now old enough to walk and talk, could feel the negative energy and vocalized her distrust in him. Still, Annette remained tight in the grip of the family, church, and community.

After nine years of torment, Annette took a good look at her reality. She was full of fear, shame, and embarrassment. She constantly thought about what people would think and do if she left her second marriage. To her, the fear of judgment, abandonment, and ridicule was worse than the life she was living.

In her role as a divorce lawyer, she coached, helped, and brought the voice of reason to other women on a daily basis. She offered them all the tools, resources, counseling, and therapy that was accessible to them. Annette knew what to do, how to do it, and what the outcomes were when a woman followed through with action steps that would better their life. She knew them by heart.

The voice inside her mind and her heart spoke loudly. She could no longer ignore it. It was her turn to reach out to these resources and use them for the greater good of her life and that of her children's. She witnessed other women take back their power and fully transform their lives. She was inspired by their bravery and decided if they could do it, so could she. Annette understood at a deep level that she had to leave her marriage.

The debris of her marriages left Annette bruised in every sense of the word. Looking at her children, deeply looking within herself and her thirty-six years of life experiences, she knew the cycle was a damaging one. She also knew that, like any storm, it had an end. Like church bells on a Sunday morning, this quote rang in Annette's ears: "The devil whispered in my ear, 'You are not strong enough to withstand the storm.' Today, I whispered in the devil's ear, 'I am the storm.'"

This time it was different. This time she chose herself. She chose to leave all the broken pieces, the debris from it all, on the ground, and when she was ready, she walked away, holding the hands of her children and nothing else. She knew she could and would rebuild her life. With one foot on the ground at a time, she looked back at the wreckage, not with the sense of obligation to return but as a reminder of the storm she walked through and survived.

SAMANTHA

"My family was broken, and my heart was broken. I had three daughters, and it was up to me to take care of them. So, I did."

To this day, there are a couple of words that when spoken cause Samantha's body, mind, and heart memory to respond—sometimes with a shiver, other times with a poke. To Samantha, the words *infidelity* and *divorce* are weighted with feelings of shame, embarrassment, heartache, rejection, and sadness.

At forty, Samantha was married with three daughters. When her husband received an opportunity to change departments at work, something he said would be better for the family, Samantha had a gut feeling that something was "off." Soon, her husband was buying new clothes, spending more time away from the family, and expressing feelings of not fitting in with their lifestyle. Although she'd had that initial gut feeling, Samantha didn't see what was coming until it "slapped her in the face."

Samantha's realization that her husband was being unfaithful was earth-shattering and brought her a fair share of emotions and responses. She felt as if she were on a roller coaster with them, and in her darkest moments, she questioned her own worthiness. Infidelity is an act of betrayal, but not one done solo. There are two people in a marriage, three when it comes to cheating. In coming to terms with her own involvement, Samantha felt a new sense of despair: "Why her? Why not me? Why can't we try and work this out?"

Unfortunately, these questions came with answers that no heart wants to hear or can bear. Where there once was love, happiness, and the idea of "forever after," there was now agony and a crushed perspective of trust.

Nothing about Samantha's "new" life was easy: the complicated emotions that follow betrayal run deep, especially grief. The love she once felt so strongly for her partner was replaced with sadness and overwhelm, emotions she did her best to release through physical activity including walking and running. Exercising allowed

Samantha time to learn more about herself and to make plans for moving forward.

In trying to move forward with no real sense of direction, Samantha needed to tap into her form of grit. Inch by inch and step by step, as the saying goes, she found traction. Deep inside she knew she had two options: she could stay full of hurt and sadness or she could take this opportunity to grow, to become a better, lighter, and more positive and present version of herself.

With releasing emotions comes power. As a first step, Samantha decided to write a letter to her ex and the new HER in his life. The letter made Alanis Morissette's "You Oughta Know" sound like church music! She put the letter in their mailbox and walked away. Funny enough, Samantha found out later that the mailbox was at the wrong address. Regardless, her thoughts had been released out of her body, mind, and heart and into the universe.

Meanwhile, her girls were experiencing their own hurt. When they would get upset about their dad and his new partner, Samantha had to continue working through her own grief and trust issues while holding the girls in their pain. And she knew it was important for the girls to still have their father in their lives. Samantha struggled with the amount of energy and effort it took to "play nice" for the sake of her girls. Slowly but surely, though, through explaining to the girls what the changes in their lives were going to look like, she began to experience a new form of confidence in herself and how she was handling new situations.

Samantha realized that the only way through it all was to find her strength and courage. She knew that her girls were watching her intently and would learn from her how to heal wounds. They, too, were experiencing their own layers of trust issues and feelings of betrayal and abandonment from their parents' divorce, something Samantha fully understood.

As time passed, Samantha began getting into the flow of her new reality. Together with her girls, she found her way and built new routines; they leaned on each other for support. They became a team and worked on trying to figure it all out together.

Samantha felt a deep connection (and still does) to a quote by Rose Fitzgerald Kennedy: "It has been said, 'time heals all wounds.' I do not agree. The wounds remain. In time, the mind, protecting its sanity, covers them with scar tissue and that pain lessens. But it is never gone."

These words told Samantha that her pain would lessen over time but would remain a memory marked by a scar that no amount of time would ever erase. But she knew that words like *love*, *compassion*, *forgiveness*, *self-perseverance*, *courage*, and *dignity* would play their part in her story too. She called upon these words for support and direction each day. They were her words of affirmation. Time brings healing, but it does not erase old memories—that is the inner work of every woman scorned, inner work that takes its fair share of time and is truly dependent upon the woman's sense of self to lead the way.

YOURstory

By enduring a storm of monumental size, whether it is weather inflicted or human experience, we understand the truest version of ourselves. It is when our grit, our fight, our determination and inner power come to light. It is within the eye of the storm that you will discover yourself. While sitting in the stillness, your fear and your love will guide you to your biggest life lesson of all—everything you ever needed to know already lives within you, and that's how you survive any storm.

REFLECTION:

Think of a moment or moments in your life when you had to endure a "storm." What did your "grit" look like? How did it feel? Did/Do you recognize your own strength?

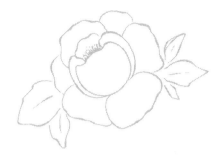

Chapter 9:
Leaning on Sisters; Believing in Self

Serendipity, synchronicities, and coincidences, I believe in them all.

An unbelievable number of serendipitous moments have happened in my life for me to lean on the trust that something bigger than my imagination is at work. At the end of May, Darryl was scheduled to write the biggest exams of his life in Ottawa. Right before he left, he took a leap of faith and applied for an orthopedic position in our hometown of Collingwood, Ontario. We knew that this was a long shot, but if he didn't apply, he would regret it. At that time it was rare for an orthopedic resident fresh out of residency to enter the working world without completing at least one fellowship, and we were scheduled to move to Toronto to begin Darryl's first one.

While he was focused on writing his exams, I was a block away in a bridesmaid's dress with our four-month-old Everett on my breast. Devon was saying, "I do," and I was there to be their witness. I had called Crystal for support with Everett and our Ottawa friends for support for Lillian. It was all hands on deck.

Shortly after we all returned home from an unforgettable weekend, fate showed up at our doorstep and our world flipped. On a Monday morning, Darryl got a message that he was scheduled for an interview for the job in Collingwood. Our house sold on the Thursday, and by Friday, Darryl was offered the position. In shock, we read the job offer aloud. Darryl, fresh out of his ortho residency, was going to be a full-time surgeon in our childhood hometown. As we took it all in, we held on to our babies and popped open a bottle of champagne. We might not have been ready for this jump, but at one of my favorite sounds in the world, the popping of a champagne cork, we said a toast to new beginnings and called our families with the news that after fourteen years, we were "coming home."

Following the fast flow of change, with one step in front of the other and full trust that it would all work out, we had twenty days to make the change from moving to Toronto to moving to Collingwood. When you only have a short window of opportunity, you have to make quick decisions, so we sought the help from our families to find us a home.

My parents jumped in. They bought an investment house in town, and within twenty days, we completely flipped it. Darryl's parents hosted us while the renovations took place, and meanwhile, Justin and Jayne sold their place and moved in with us when our home was complete. We were one big happy family.

It wasn't all smooth sailing, however. The assumption made by many was that it would be an easy transition for Darryl and me to move back home. We were both born and raised in the area, our families were rooted in the community, and we had several childhood friends still residing there. I knew better, though. The person I was when I left the town at eighteen and the person I was returning to it at thirty-one were not the same, and neither was our town. Our return would be as different as we were, and our adjustment would be our next big adventure.

The first six months were somewhat rocky. I had an old high school acquaintance reach out to me, asking if I'd meet her for a lunch date. On arriving at the café, I realized that not everyone had changed. After a long pause and awkward reintroduction, she made her intentions clear: "I just wanted to see if you know, made it or not. See how you aged." Stunned by her comment, my mind flooded with doubts about whether we had made the right decision to move "home."

A phone call with Shannon recentered me. She was the voice of reason using our "snowball" theory. When you start off, the snowball is small. As you continue to roll, the snowball grows, takes shape, and forms. So keep rolling and go with the snowfall. I found comfort in her words of support and encouragement to give this new phase more time.

Shortly after that experience, I ran into yet another high school friend, Jen Flint, or "Flinty." Her embrace was warm, loving, and familiar. She was out shopping with her little guy, who's just a couple months younger than Everett. We instantly reconnected, exchanged numbers, and I let out a huge sigh of relief. I had rediscovered a friend.

I also reconnected with Sabrina, Darryl's first cousin. We had been friends throughout the years, and when her girls were little,

I would make special trips home to spend time with them. We'd have dates to the beach, do shopping trips, have dress-up parties, and read bedtime stories. I had been in their life since they were babies. And now that I was back home and had children of my own, Sabrina's girls reversed the support and became our family babysitters. This came in handy when I was focused on integration plus my usual "get shit done" list. It also ensured that I had more quality time together with Sabrina. Our friendship blossomed into soul-sister status.

Little by little, I started making connections with old friends who introduced me to new friends. One day a lady who worked with Darryl invited us over for dinner. The topic of running came up in conversation, and she mentioned that she would be leading a run clinic. Excited, I signed up. And in doing so, I met the most amazing group of women. They were "go" women. They wanted what I wanted—their cake and all the bites too! We took on hill training together and ran up and down hills for breakfast! I hadn't known how powerful my legs and body were until these ladies challenged me to find out. The encouragement we found in each other was contagious.

Soon, we were socializing at each other's houses (both with all our kids and without) and searching for the next adventure to take on. My children were thriving because I was thriving. They were making friends and having playdates, and so was I. Even the conversations we were having, mom to mom and woman to woman, were growth focused. We did not sit around bitching about the things we didn't have or gossiping over mindless bullshit. We were engaged in each other's worlds in a positive way. I was making connections with women who inspired me and lifted my energy to a level I had been longing for.

In being surrounded by these women, women who focused on being the best version of themselves, I felt a strong nudge to return to school. I decided to follow a childhood passion: interior design. For each apartment or house I had lived in, I'd loved the process of taking a blank canvas and completely redesigning the layout and colors and bringing in different textures. And in thinking back to my childhood, I remembered playing in my dad's showroom and creating mood boards without really understanding what I was doing. I'd always had an eye for design, and at this point in my life, learning more about it was only something to gain.

There is power in saying yes to something that nudges you from your very core, as it sends out vibrations that opens doors to other opportunities. The love and support you give and receive when you belong to a village of women and their families was in full bloom for us, and our energy was glowing.

Running in these circles, I noticed that more and more conversations were becoming centered around creating activities just for women. Additionally, some of my mom friends were returning to work or taking on new positions as consultants and entrepreneurs. This was a world that intrigued me, so I decided to throw a party, a "Bubbles" party. To me, the idea was simple: I would clear out my house, order in charcuterie boards, and provide lots of champagne (a.k.a. the "bubbles!").

Right before the Bubbles party was to happen, a conversation with my cousin's wife, a new consultant for a bag company, sparked another idea in me. She had expressed that she needed an audience for her bag parties. It was divine timing. I told her to bring her product and set it up in my dining room, and that I'd give her a window of time during the party to deliver the story of why she believed in it. It was the first collaboration of many that these Bubbles parties would see.

That first night kicked off with more than forty women attending with their best friends and sisters. The volume of chatter and music increased by the hour, and so did the energy of my house. Women were laughing, clinking glasses, telling stories, and engaging in conversation. And something magical happened. A light turned on inside me. I had a purpose.

I was finally part of a community that I had been wanting to have for so long, and I could share it with others! I had the house to hold the Bubbles parties, the ideas to expand on them, and the connections with other leading ladies in the business world who needed an audience for their products and businesses! Before long, one Bubbles party turned into a spring event, then a yoga, Zumba, and athletic apparel party, then a jewelry and breast cancer party. When I wasn't attending mommy-and-me playdates, completing schoolwork, or training for my next race, I was planning the next Bubbles party! I finally felt as if I was in full bloom.

A Sunday afternoon in late spring brought sudden change. Oh, the dualities of life. My parents-in-law were visiting and shared the news of Sabrina's ongoing cancer prognosis. Over the past couple years, the word *cancer* had darkened her doorstep, and with each recurrence, she mustered up the strength to endure the treatment plans and all the drugs and surgeries that came with them. This was something we knew was a part of her daily life, and ours too. We were involved in all the light and dark moments of a family going through the cancer journey.

When her girls were in school, Sabrina and I went on day dates and talked about everything together, including the hard topics like death that can make some people uncomfortable. By this time, I had graduated with my interior design degree and had hosted several parties, and I'd decided that returning to school for event planning was my next step in life. Sabrina loved hearing all about the schoolwork and what my next big thing was going to be. Her treatments were coming to an end and her energy was improving, and I wanted to celebrate her cancer victory. With the holiday season approaching, it was the perfect time to host the biggest Bubbles party yet.

It was to be a holiday market that would showcase twelve female-led businesses. There would be a fashion show from a local fashion house, an inspirational speaker, and the notorious dance party, of course. To level it up one more notch, I asked every lady attending to pay it forward by bringing an unwrapped toy, food donation, and/or the monetary value of it. All proceeds would be donated to our local women's shelter and food bank. Details like this mattered to me.

That Bubbles party saw 100 ladies walk and then dance through my home. Before the night took off, I popped a special bottle of champagne and said a private toast to Sabrina and her daughter Lora. It was a toast to health, friendship, and a shit ton of fun we were going to have. Our future was looking bright. I then refilled my glass and joined my team on my staircase for a speech that would open up the rest of the night to dancing and celebrating.

"To all the ladies here in this house! Each and every one of you has a reason for being here. You might have needed a girls' night, a night away from your children and/or partner. You might have been simply curious. Maybe your reason is to let go of something that weighs on you and needs a little support from friends or you love champagne and want to dance! Whatever the reason, tonight we support you and that need, and we thank you for coming! I'll end 2018 with a quote from Maya Angelou. She said, 'I've learned that people will forget what you said, people will forget what you did, but people will never forget how you made them feel.' So if you leave this night feeling that love, support, and happiness, that glow you get from your girlfriends and a couple bottles of champagne, then I'd say we did our bit!"

Three days later, the house was cleaned and put back together, pictures and stories were posted, and all was right in the world. Everyone's hangover was cured, but one. Sabrina, still feeling ill and not able to recover from a migraine, went to see her doctor and called me directly with the results. Taking in the news, I froze. I couldn't respond. I could hear her words but could not process fast enough to get out any words of my own. Her cancer had metastasized to her brain. It was back, and with a vengeance.

Sitting with the news and the projected "time frame," I felt like my color disappeared. I could no longer see the bright future I'd just toasted to, and I couldn't stop thinking about her daughters. I stopped everything. No more parties, no more events. My new priority was focusing on the time we could spend together with her and her girls.

On one of our day dates, Sabrina and I spent some much-needed girl time together with lunch, window shopping, and a visit to a tarot card reader. While at lunch, Sabrina brought up my schooling. She wanted to focus on positive topics, nothing heavy or sad. So I shared with her all the details of my upcoming business idea. I wanted to start an event planning company that would spark joy and girl time in every celebration I hosted.

She listened so intently. She nodded her head and took in the details, and when the moment was right, she laughed and said, "Oh, Ashley, it is so much bigger than that." She then shared with me a vision of my future that only she could see as a result of our shared experiences and the reality that they were coming to an end. She knew the journey I would go on. She spoke of my purpose, of my finding myself, and all that was ahead for her girls, my daughter, and the women who attended my events and Bubbles parties. Although her vision was beyond my sight, I trusted her wisdom and leaned into it with a deep love for my friend, my soul sister. She saw me and thus, I saw myself.

HERstory

EMILY

"After a lifetime of searching, I know that when I teach or practice yoga, I am seen, valued, and heard; most importantly, so are my students. They see the light in me and together, we belong."

To belong is a human need; it starts the second you are born and lasts a lifetime. When you belong to YOU, truly, unconditionally, authentically, and undeniably, you belong everywhere you go and with anyone who accompanies you.

Deep within Emily there was a special kind of soul, a healing soul that knew the many faces of anxiety, depression, and mental illness. All throughout her life, she'd been witness to her mother's, father's, and sister's struggles with mental health, so she recognized when she, herself, began experiencing anxiety. Right around the time her second child was born, Emily started feeling anxious. She knew she had a good job, a great house and partner, and friendships she enjoyed, and she deeply loved being a mother to her daughter and new son. But with all that was wonderful in her life, she still felt as if something were missing. She wasn't depressed, but she wasn't happy, something that caused her concern. She worried that she would suffer in the same ways that her family members had and wondered what she could do about it. So she went into self-help mode: she read self-love/self-help books and practiced deeper explorations into her soul. She was introduced to yoga and meditation, and during her first yoga class, it was as if a switch turned on and she could see what she was missing from her life right in front of her.

Emily desperately didn't want the cycle of mental health struggles to repeat with her children. On the mat that day, with tears in her eyes and memories of her own childhood flooding her thoughts, Emily realized that yoga would be her entrance into healing herself. This discovery led Emily to attend many classes and then into a yoga teaching training program.

"My family did not understand how much yoga changed, helped, and encouraged me to be the different one. I realized that if it can empower and heal me, then I need to do this for as many people as I can. I knew that there was not only one answer to mental health. I focused on healing others and inadvertently, it healed me."

When her son turned one, Emily returned to work at a cancer center, a place with the sole mission of supporting, aiding, and providing treatment, love, and hope to people battling all different forms of cancer. To other staff members and work buddies, Emily shared her dreams and ambitions of becoming a yoga instructor, a job that to many was not attainable or a smart decision. They couldn't understand why she would leave a job with a great pension, job security, longevity, and to them, purpose. But to Emily, the job did not fulfill her soul.

During her shifts, Emily talked with patients. In these conversations, they all expressed messages of what living meant to them, and not one ever mentioned their pension. They spoke of regrets and of their own grief about living with and dying from a disease that knows no prejudices. In these interactions, Emily was frequently reminded of her own desire to live a life of purpose—to live every day feeling humble and grateful, and to be in service for the greater good.

To add to the heaviness of her shifts, Emily had a new manager who brought down her team and bullied several of the staff, including Emily. Many times, Emily would find excuses not to go into work, and every shift sparked feelings of anxiousness. She would cry in her car, in the bathroom while at work, and then again on her way home. She would ask herself, "How can someone make you feel so small, so insignificant?" Her answer: "They can't."

Emily knew it was time to make a change. Her heart, soul, and life depended upon it. She created a vision board and declared to the Universe, to her higher self, and to her friends and her family what she wanted and what she was going after.

"I want more in this life. I want a deep, meaningful, leadership-inspired, create-my-own-path kind of life. I am showing my children that you can be what you want to be and that taking care of yourself first helps you take care of your family. You have to do the work, but you are worth the work. Practice, meditation, teaching—I am learning and taking my teachings with me every time my students and I step onto our mats. I want to lead the charge to better inner health."

Her true belonging would be found within her inner knowing that she was born to inspire, to be a guide to healing. She was the soft and friendly voice of a teacher whose main goal in life was not to merely survive, but to thrive internally and externally. She felt her belonging during yoga teacher training. She had friends and was part of a community, and when she returned home to her family, she returned with a sense of inclusivity, purpose, alignment, and energy! She had found her true calling. She felt it and then lived it.

KRISTAL

"I am learning to listen to my own body—the movement, its feelings, all of it. Intuitively, I did this before when I was pregnant with Emma, but after reaching my heaviest weight and my darkest hours, I knew that I needed to do more than listen. I would make this change for ME and for her; the rest will fall into place."

At a very young age, Kristal knew the difference between small girls and big girls. Around the time when she was understanding what her female body was made of, she was also discovering the connection between her body and her worth. The perspective of what she thought she "should" be came from overhearing the conversations between other women, all the girls at school, and the strong presence of the media and social norms.

Starting around the age of thirteen and continuing into her adult life, Kristal was consciously aware of her fluctuating body weight. When she lost weight, she heard positive comments, uplifting praises, and encouragement from others. When she put on weight, she heard silence and felt disapproval when eating in public.

After giving birth to her daughter, Emma, Kristal experienced postpartum depression, which lead to a period of weight gain and her darkest time of life. Kristal began noticing comments that family members, friends, and even strangers were making about Emma: "She's soooo small" and then "Look how big she's grown." Comments about Emma's size triggered Kristal, and after having an honest conversation with her husband, Andrew, about her struggles over her body issues, they decided that they wanted to give Emma a different type of environment in which to grow up.

Kristal and Andrew established some boundaries about how people spoke about food, health, and body size around Emma. Kristal spoke to Emma's teachers, dance instructors, and family members, but despite her best efforts, Emma, a healthy and active seven-year-old, came home in tears one day saying, "I don't look like the other girls. I'm fat."

There it was: the dreaded word. Hearing Emma call herself "fat" caused Kristal to have a flashback to her own youth:

"I remembered trying to fit into prom dresses and being made fun of by boys for being what they deemed 'fat.' I didn't want Emma to have to go through those hurtful things or to feel like what made her worthy was her weight or size. She's worked so extremely hard as a dancer, and I didn't want her to lose her passion because she felt that she didn't fit within the body norms that have been presented to her by society. These harmful ingrained beliefs do their damage and have the ability to stay with you."

All the time, energy, and effort Kristal had put into changing her own mindset about her body weight and physical health had not prepared her for the moment when her little girl made her first comment about her own weight. For Kristal, after a lifetime of looking into the mirror and seeing her weight first, it was at that moment she realized that her call to action was no longer just about what she wanted for herself. Together with her husband, Kristal spoke to Emma about the strength needed for dancing, the muscles she'd developed, and how good it feels to move your body. They discussed Emma's women role models, and how she did not pay attention to their size. They also spoke about the dancers at Emma's studio, all of whom had different body frames.

After a lengthy conversation with Emma, Kristal returned to her room, looked in the mirror, and cried. She felt like she'd failed her daughter. She was at a heavier weight, and she believed she had given up on her body and herself. At some point, she had just stopped caring. Kristal wanted to put in the work to realign with a healthy body weight. She wanted to find the strength to do it so she would be in tune with her body, and herself, again.

Kristal's mother suggested gastric bypass surgery as an option to investigate. It was an extreme, life-altering decision, and Kristal felt some discomfort over the idea of surgery—why would she do that to herself? But she wanted to make a sustainable change, so she took a couple days to think about it and came to a new perspective. This was her beginning.

Kristal started doing research. One of her lifelong friends had recently had the surgery, had completely changed her lifestyle, and was now celebrating her successes. Her friend was glowing, and not just because she lost the weight but because she was living her best life with energy, confidence, and self-love. Kristal's aunt, who'd also undergone the surgery, was also dancing up a storm in her life and had the energy to do it. Kristal understood that the results were not the same for everyone, nor would it be an easy transformation. It would be so much more than just having the surgery: Kristal would have to change her mindset, understand her triggers and trauma, and reinvent her relationship with food.

Kristal established the goals of being active, healthy, and excited about life for herself and, most importantly, her daughter. She scheduled her first appointment where it was determined that she was an ideal candidate for the procedure. She was introduced to a dietitian, a fitness instructor, and a physiologist, the team that would work with her physical, mental, and emotional health both before and after the surgery.

Kristal felt an immediate connection with her dietitian. She didn't judge Kristal, and she gave her all the tools she needed to help her on her journey. Her kindness made Kristal feel supported and at ease. She also felt supported by family, friends, and Emma, all of whom cheered her on and were excited for her in her journey to health and wellness.

Andrew, however, was not. He'd had his own journey of physical pain and surgeries and knowing what Kristal was going to undergo scared him. Time after time, he would say to her, "You need to show me that you can eat healthy and keep exercising and then I will support you." In hearing these words, Kristal internalized that she wasn't good enough, that she had not tried hard enough and was taking the easy way out.

This was the turning point for Kristal. She was not having this surgery and making these lifestyle changes for him, for society, or for the two sections in the clothing department. She was doing this for HER—she was dedicated to *herself*. With that knowledge, she spoke up.

"This is my body and my life, and nobody is going to tell me what I can or cannot do. I never want Emma to be held back by anyone. I want her to vocalize what is best for her and her life, and I will show her how. I will be getting this surgery. I would love to have you by my side, but if you aren't able to put your fears and issues aside, that will not change my decision. This is about ME; it is my decision to make."

Kristal's determined stance made a difference. Andrew started asking questions and taking an interest in the surgery, and Kristal knew he was now supporting her decision. She also knew that having her support systems and people ready for post surgery was just as important as the team that was preparing her for it.

The first twenty-four hours of recovery were the hardest. Kristal was so sick that she had moments when she thought she would pass out. Thankfully, her support system was in place to help. But despite having this help, Kristal knew that it was up to her to get back on her feet—she had to dig deep for the determination and fight to heal. She had to relearn her body's needs and what fueled her and what did not.

Slowly, Kristal began to bounce back. Soon, her learning curve was not only focused on what her body needed but also about what she needed for her inner healing. Societal norms, judgments, and pressures were all still out there, but Kristal worked hard to understand that they were unrealistic and did not represent her as a person. She switched off the noise, listened deeply to herself, and became fully aligned and committed to her own healing journey.

As Kristal's positive mindset about her self-worth continued to develop, her relationships experienced their own growth. Her marriage felt stronger and more secure and communicative. And with Emma, Kristal was proud to have her daughter witness her go through something hard—to work through the discomfort and dedicate herself to self-love and healing—and come out the other side transformed and full of life. She was proud that Emma saw her discover all the layers of herself including her goals, strengths, and aspirations.

Kristal's journey from shame to confidence is one that she will forever walk. She knows that as she continues on this path, she has the support from her family and friends. Most importantly, however, she knows what she is capable of achieving because she believes in herself.

YOURstory

Having a support system, a community to depend on, is important, but believing in oneself is vital. It is when you truly focus inward on your strengths and ambitions that you can see who you are and what you are capable of, and having people support you in this growth along the way is worth celebrating. But you are the one who makes the decisions to act and react, to answer the call. You have to show up for yourself.

REFLECTION:

Recall a pinnacle moment, light or dark, in your life. Did you have a support system? Did YOU show up for yourself?

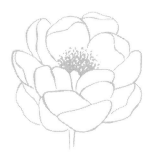

Chapter 10:
Loss and Heartache

For months, I would have a recurring dream, one where I was in Sabrina's home in an incredibly long hallway. In slow motion yet with the loud sound of my heart racing, I was running down this hallway that had no end in sight. Running toward me were Sabrina's daughters, yet we would never quite reach each other. Each time I had the dream, it became more evident that something was lurking. I could feel it but could do nothing to stop it.

The school year was coming to an end and Darryl, the kids, and I were packing and getting ready for a trip to Ottawa to visit friends and attend our annual summer get-togethers. Just before we left, I told Sabrina that we had a whole summer of activities to do together and that I would be right back so to not go anywhere. She smiled, agreed, and said, "I love you, girl."

I couldn't settle or sleep the entire time we were gone. My worries and nudges that I needed to get home kept getting stronger. I could feel the pull and the distance of every kilometer. I tried my best to be present with everyone, but I wasn't. I knew without knowing that I needed to return to Collingwood.

My sense of urgency brought us home early on a Sunday morning, and my first course of action was to call Sabrina and make a date. A soul sister knows you from the inside out; she knows what you need and what to say. Upon hearing Sabrina's voice, I could tell right away that a shift had occurred while we were gone and although she didn't get into the details on the phone, she told me that she had reserved the next day for us to spend together.

That Monday, we had the perfect lunch date. Sabrina's partner and their eldest daughter, Lora, joined us. We ate deep-fried pickles, burgers, fries, and salads and laughed at old stories while dreaming of new adventures. After lunch, as Sabrina and I were in the car, she asked if we could make a stop, a short visit to see her Aunt Elaine, my mother-in-law. During this time Sabrina shared with me her plans for our summer adventures with the girls. She said I was the right woman with the right energy to carry out these plans for her.

She made three simple requests that I promised to keep:

For Lora, run up the hill with her at the Summit 700 Blue Mountain Race.

For Lainey, take her to Canada's Wonderland and on her first roller coaster—the really big one.

For Livi, spend quality time with her! Plan a girls' weekend away with all the girls and stay in a hotel.

Nodding my head, I said yes and made her a promise to see it through. While helping her walk up to her doorway, we laughed about big butts and getting back into shape with our liquid salad recipe (our version of the Caesar cocktail) and confirmed our plans for the week: on Wednesday I would pick up Livi after camp and then on Saturday I had the big Summit 700 race with Lora. I hugged her goodbye and said, "See you Wednesday!" You don't know until you know and when you know, you can't unknow what you know.

Two days later it was perfect weather for a trip to the beach with my girlfriends and all our kids. We headed out, and I couldn't help but feel that something about the day felt slow and out of place. As I unpacked the car on our arrival, my phone rang, and with the sound of the voice on the other end, time stopped. I looked out into the big bay of dark blue water and lost my breath. Little sips of air entered my lips, tears rolled down my cheeks, and my heart sank to a new level of despair. I walked right into the water. There, waves brushed against my legs and I swayed back and forth, lulling myself with the rhythm of the tide.

I couldn't look at anyone. Something told this group of women that my world was twirling, and their instant reaction was to hold the space around me still, calm, and secure. They took care of my children and didn't know that their mere presence brought air back into my lungs and grounded my feet.

My heart knew one thing while my brain was already processing my next steps and how to respond. Time moved at a snail's pace, and it was as though every breath I took moved the waves of the water and the clouds in the sky. "Just breathe, Ashley," my inner voice whispered.

It was time to go; it was time to connect with the girls and their mother. My sister backed me up by packing and loading up my babies for whatever was to come next and for however long it would take.

In the car with Livi, and en route to get her sisters, I told her that her mother's love is the forever kind; that the moment Sabrina had known she was expecting Livi, she'd created an unbreakable bond with her that would be held together throughout all of time, a bond that not even death could break. I knew that it was going to be one of the hardest days of her life.

We walked into the sterile building and prepared ourselves to be greeted with the uncertainty of time with their mother. Only that time was important, and it wasn't anything we could control. My mantra, "Body in motion, stays in motion," repeated in my thoughts.

Seeing Sabrina lying in her hospital bed, without her wig and hooked up to machines, caused my heart to drop to a level I had never experienced before. I had never been witness to someone I held so dear in the final hours of life. Everyone had their own time with her, gentle moments of gratitude, love, and tenderness, and when it was my turn, I held her hand and whispered, "Hey, girl, I am right here. I love you, sister." Under her breath and in a voice so soft that only I could hear, she said, "Hold them." Understanding the gravity of these last words, I made her the promise: "Always."

The night was long, far too long for the girls. We decided to take them home to my place for some rest with the plan to return in the morning. When we left the hospital, we walked right into the warmest, gentlest summer rain. It was beautiful. On our drive home, the girls requested that we listen to Jasmine Thompson and her rendition of "You Are My Sunshine," a song that to this day still makes me weep.

I fell asleep that night listening to the quiet rain and was awoken the next morning by the sun's rays. I took the opportunity in the peacefulness to seek my own comfort and called Flinty while sipping on my coffee. Her voice settled my nerves. There was no sense of urgency or rush, only ease and stillness. Then, instinctually, we all knew when it was time to return to the hospital.

My ability to "hold"—hold back my tears, hold strong for the girls, hold my breath, hold all of it—started to collapse as I entered Sabrina's room and heard her breathing. Overnight, it had turned to a death rattle. I lost my grip, exited the room, and found a quiet place in the garden area of the first floor. There, surrounded by flowers, garden benches, and statues, I called my parents in tears. My dad spoke first: "Baby, it will be all over soon. We love you. Be strong." My mom then added: "You've got this, Ashley, now go to her." At that moment, a circle of butterflies danced around me, and I knew that Sabrina was gone.

I ran as though I had wings! Up the flight of stairs and around the nurses' station, I skidded into the hallway, the incredibly long hallway where I saw Lora and Livi running toward me, stopping only once they reached my arms. As I held them, I looked up and saw the most beautiful fuchsia paper-mache butterfly on Sabrina's doorway.

Months prior, Lora and I had registered for Blue Mountain's Summit 700, a challenging trail run for anyone. A day after her mother passed away, Lora, a committed athlete in any sport she took on, asked if we could still run it. She wanted to see it through and told me that Sabrina, just a week before, had said she would be there to watch it. "Okay, let's do this," I said, remembering my promise to her mother. I knew the race would be tough on both of us, and not just because of the 6 km trail up the mountain. It was taking place on the same day as Sabrina's viewing and final goodbye at the funeral home.

In preparation for the run, I called Joanna, my forever running partner, and asked her to pick up our running bibs and to sign Lora and me in for the Saturday morning race. Joanna went the extra step. Unbeknownst to me, she called our friend Amanda, and together they made the split-second decision to join us. They registered, picked up matching shirts, and arranged to run the race with us.

Completely exhausted, I geared up and was "ready" to run. I was very present to what was happening around me; I would just be going through the process. While driving up to the mountain, Joanna pulled off to the side of the road where Amanda was waiting: a planned stop for her but a secret to me. Amanda hopped in the car and in her humorous way said, "Let's get this show on the road. It's only 6 km uphill . . . how bad could it be?"

Leading up to this moment, I had been too occupied with everything else to even give myself time to take in what I was feeling, nevermind cry. With Joanna and Amanda in the car, I cried. Here they were, my two girlfriends, flying in to rescue me. In front of them I could be vulnerable and release the "hold." They showed up! They put everything on hold, knowing what the adventure was, and they showed up for me in a way that I did not expect. I was floored and overwhelmed with such admiration, love, and support.

At the beginning of the race, Lora and I looked directly up the hill we were about to run. I have no idea where our energy came from. Less than three days prior to this moment, I had stood beside my soul sister's hospital bed and promised to care for her girls. And here I was about to run a race up the mountain with one of them.

As we ran, there were many times we lost our breath and struggled to keep going in the hot sun. My body was overheated, in shock, and on the edge of falling apart. At one point I bowed my head, shook it, and with a simple look up and a glance right into Joanna's eyes, without words, I told her all the fears of defeat in my head. She grabbed my hand and said, "You've got her and we've got you. You can do this, Ashley. Keep going." A soft voice then spoke loudly enough for me to hear it: "Just breathe." I regrouped. Nodding to the girls, I took Lora's hand and we trudged through the forest with Amanda and Joanna right behind us

Minutes later, my mom, a woman who does not run or hike, somehow found the exact spot where we would be exiting the forest trail. Her timing was perfect. She was completely aligned with us. As I ran out of the tree line, there she was with my dad. They, too, had shown up for me. An embrace of my mom's love gave me strength I'd longed for my whole life. I could have stayed in her arms forever, but I knew we were in a race and that it was time to let go and keep running. I was hit with a surge of energy that can only be described as coming from the power of love, support, and guidance from above. Lora and I finished that race together. I had fulfilled my first promise.

Shortly afterward, one of Sabrina's friends offered to set up a day at Canada's Wonderland, a theme park in Toronto, for Lainey and me. It would be an opportunity for me to fulfill another promise. Lainey had never been on a roller coaster, and the first one she wanted to ride just so happened to be the biggest and fastest with the steepest drop. Standing at the bottom of the ride and looking up, I said, "Holy shit!" Nevertheless, this was the one she wanted to ride, so we were going to do it. As we prepared ourselves for the drop, I held Lainey's hand and said, "Enjoy!" We fell into the rush, the swoop, and the loop-de-loops. I couldn't breathe; I couldn't even close my eyes. My hand lost its grip and slipped out of hers, never to reconnect. This ride completely took my breath away! But I rode it with Lainey, and we spent the day together full of laughter and adrenaline. Promise number two was fulfilled.

To keep my third promise to Sabrina, her friends and I organized a full weekend sleepover for all of us plus Livi and my daughter, Lillian. One of the ladies suggested that we, as a team, do the Cancer Mud Run, the Mudmoiselle. Excited, we made T-shirts, got matching bandannas, braided our hair, and wore long socks that said "fierce" up the sides. We were Sabrina's warriors, and we were united. At the beginning of the race, we took a knee and declared aloud and in unison a pledge to sisterhood and a promise to fight for the survivors. Then we swore to remember our sister in the sky.

I had done several obstacle runs before this one and thought I knew what to expect. This run, though, was different. This time

I was encouraging Sabrina's girls to keep moving forward and was running with a group of grieving women who drew their strength from each other. We ran, climbed, went through a pond, and laughed. When we celebrated our victory, I also celebrated completing my third promise. There was only one more thing to do: "hold them." And I would. My promise was forever.

Sabrina's friends and I had no idea what would come next, only that we had three girls who needed us to keep showing up. I was not prepared for what that would mean and had no idea just how hard it would be. Grief is one thing to experience for yourself, but to be a firsthand witness to the grief of the three girls and their father, that was another. I began immediately responding to anything they needed—clothes, haircuts, an all-hours referee for their fights—my heart was invested in it all. I was their warrior, a true defender, and I was in way over my head. It was all-consuming and exhausting.

In the process of doing everything, I lost everything. I stop listening to my heart. Along with my own grief, my fears, insecurities, and ego took over. A fight between the girls during their first Christmas holiday without their mom did us all in. I snapped. Instead of being an adult and choosing to walk away, I raised my voice and got right into it with Lainey. For six months I had put every ounce of myself into being available for them. I hadn't even begun to process my own loss. Lainey screamed, I screamed. She slammed doors, and I melted to the kitchen floor in complete surrender. Everyone was hurting, and we didn't have the words to connect with each other.

The walls between us grew high, and I didn't have the energy to climb them. So, I let her go. I may have won the battle, but I definitely lost the war. In losing Lainey, I became fearful of losing the other two girls as well. Without fully realizing it, I became even more overprotective of Lora; I went into defense mode and held on too tight.

A crack in the surface occurred when I realized that grief is far more complex than I had originally believed. I was learning lessons about grief, conflict, and how people react during dark times. And that grief is not limited to just losing someone to death, it can be losing someone over a conversation that went wrong. Miscommunication over an event took hold, and instead of confronting the issue, we had ghosting behavior, walked away, and blamed; we had the limiting belief that "it's everyone else's fault but mine." All these fear-based responses landed instead of leaning into the place where love once lived.

I started experiencing recurring flashbacks to miscommunications and conflicts between friends I'd had throughout my life. A tsunami of deep-seated family conflicts and memories of fight, flight, or freeze moments flooded me. I remembered fears and insecurities of not being accepted, of not belonging with friend groups that I walked away from. I was caught in a recurring pattern passed down to me from a generation that swept problems under rugs, spoke about each other but not to each other, and perfected the art of ghosting.

During this time of grieving, I'd opened a wound and was bleeding out. I sat in my grief of not just losing my soul sister but also in every relationship that I'd walked away from due to my own fears of conflict and confusion over what love is. And thus, I reverted to what I knew about dealing with problems: my voice got big, I yelled and screamed, then I walked away. I became silent. It was a complete removal, with no explanation, no words, no closure, and no connection or contact with the other person—a tactic that hurts for a longer period of time and leaves the other person in no-man's land. To me, the silent removal was by far the most damaging kind of conflict response, one that I also knew too well. I hung on so tight out of fear of losing that I ended up suffocating more than Lora and our relationship. And in doing this, I lost everything. A true fall from grace.

HERstory

MAGDA

"I have to go on the journey. I don't want to hurt anyone's feelings, but I need them, as well as myself, to know that I need to go through this. I have always pushed it away and now, my body, my heart, my everything is hurting. Now is the time to heal."

Dedicated, smart, a natural leader and problem solver, multitasker, and perfectionist, Magda is the woman who gets everything done, and to a level of perfection. Every ounce of her is put into building a life for her children, a life that never lets them second-guess their safety, love, and unity. Her family and children are her first priority. Magda's strive for perfection is wrapped up in her comfort knowing that her children will never live the life she did.

At the young age of seven, Magda said goodbye to her mother, little sister, and grandparents, plus her community, home, friends, and life, and left Poland to start a new chapter in Canada with her father. She knew that one day her mother and sister would join them, but for a little girl, time was irrelevant. All she felt at that time was the loss of security, love, nurture, and family. She had no idea that her childhood was over and that her new role would soon be defined. She could not have known that she would build a barrier of protection, her new companion, out of a need for control and perfectionism. These would become like an invisible cloak she wore at home.

Magda and her father moved into her grandfather's duplex with him. Also living there were her mother's brother and his wife. The power struggle between Magda's father and her mother's father, Magda's grandfather, began the moment they moved in. To Magda's father, living under the influence and rules of his father-in-law was not positive or pleasant.

The shock of their new living environment placed a heavy toll on her father, a man who when in Poland was respected, joyful, and secure within his family. Soon, Magda's father began drinking alcohol, a bad habit that was influenced and encouraged by Magda's grandfather and uncle who were struggling alcoholics. Magda, just a little girl who loved to sing, play, and dance, was living in a space she knew was unsafe, and she was there without her mother or any support. When fights between the men grew out of control and became dangerous, it was Magda who had to call the police—a call she made numerous times.

When at home, Magda did her best to keep the peace. She kept quiet and didn't cause any trouble, stress, or heartache. She didn't want to burden anyone with her mere existence. It was at school that Magda found her sanctuary, serenity, joy, and comfort. There, she shone. She learned quickly and soaked up all the lessons, language, tools, and help she could. The praise from her teachers and the fun with the other children gave her the fuel to thrive and a new sense of security. She made friends and often wanted to be a part of their home life and structure. Magda was always careful that her own home life did not overlap with the life she had at school and with her friends. Keeping the two worlds separate was always the goal.

As she grew up, Magda became an expert at hiding her home life. To the outside world, her life seemed perfect, and controlling these two "lives" and keeping them separate was Magda's way of keeping balance. By the time her mother and sister arrived in Canada, Magda had well-established systems that kept the chaos at bay. When Magda turned eleven, her second sister was born, and her role in the family changed—she was now expected to help raise her sisters and keep them safe from their alcoholic relatives and the battles. Magda felt like she had double duty: she had to keep up the picture-perfect image she worked incredibly hard to create while at school, and while she was at home, she fought to maintain peace.

"There was no safety—the house was always unpredictable. Nothing was sturdy; nothing was grounded. I never knew what I was coming home to: Was it going to be a good day or a bad day? And the bad days were drunken messes—DUIs, fighting, etc. It was a toxic house. I constantly worried about everyone else and feared being a burden, so I never asked anyone for help. I did everything by myself, partly due to trust issues and partly because I feared that if I did become a burden, I would change the relationships or cause heartache, discomfort, and stress. To me, that was worse."

Magda was twenty-seven years old when her father got his third DUI and was detained for twenty-four hours in jail. At the time, Magda had finished university, was living on her own, and was engaged to the love of her life. She had successfully removed herself from the toxic house and had taken on more positive roles. But one phone call changed everything.

While detained, her father had attempted suicide and was now in the hospital hooked up to machines to keep him alive long enough for him to recover. Magda immediately fell back into the roles she'd held while living at home: she once again became the controlled problem solver and family defender. She took a deep breath and handled the situation on autopilot. She settled her mother, calmed her sisters, and spoke to the police officers and doctors. As she restored order, she plotted the next steps as "here we go again" played in her mind. Magda registered her father for rehab, gathered his medication, and drove him to the rehabilitation facility herself. Then for weeks she traveled back and forth to visit him and receive updates from the doctors.

In one of her visits, which she fit in between working two jobs and making wedding preparations, the storm cleared for a moment and Magda's father told her he loved her. It was only the second time she'd ever heard him say it. But upon his release from rehab, Magda's father sadly returned to his habitual behaviors and Magda's anxiety heightened once again. This time, however, Magda realized at last that she could not save her father, nor was it her responsibility to. She was not his parent, she was his child, and it was time for that distinction to be made.

Magda threw herself into the future she wanted and created for herself. She got married, started her career, and had her first son. And with the birth of two more children, Magda's dedication to her family grew. She worked long, hard hours and was fully dedicated to everything she touched. And once again, to the outside world, she was perfect—the perfect mother, wife, friend, and community member. Other women often commented on and pointed out all the ways that Magda succeeded in everything she did, but little did they know that she was breaking inside. She slept fitfully, and she was riddled with anxiety over memories of her childhood when her perfection existed as a way to control her unpredictable and chaotic home life. To Magda, her "drug" of choice was control—she needed to control every aspect of everything, and when she couldn't she'd spin . . . she'd keep herself so busy that she wouldn't have to think about or deal with what was hidden inside her.

When her oldest son turned eight, the age Magda had been when her whole world had changed, she began experiencing tsunami waves of emotions: anger, resentment, fear, and grief—grief over a lost childhood. Her body and heart ached for what hadn't been.

Now in her forties, Magda is working on healing. She wants women to know that what you see on the outside isn't always the pretty and perfect package it appears to be. She did not have the love, security, and comfort she longed for as a child, and she now knows that she needs to bring her deep-seated traumas to the surface. But she does not want to be defined by what she has endured. Magda believes that her redemption is providing her children with a profound sense of safety and a deep knowing that they are loved. Her "rising from the ashes" story has begun.

EDIE

"My parents encouraged me to do something with my degree, while my soul was pulling me toward health, healing, and yoga. It was a transition period in my life. If I hadn't taken it, changed direction, and truly listened to my heart, I wouldn't have reconnected with the things that brought me joy, nor would I have been able to be there for my mother in the last moments of her life."

Edie was working at a firm when she felt an inner calling that changed her life forever. She had given her job a solid try and learned a ton about her own resilience, reserve, boundaries, and self-worth, but while on a yoga/meditation retreat in Bali, she realized that the corporate lifestyle was not for her. So she quit her job, gave up her lease, and with no clear plan, she answered the call from her heart and moved home.

Little did Edie know that she would be put to the test when her mother's health started to decline. Ruth, Edie's mom, was the light in the world for so many people. She was a well-known, loved, and respected community leader who was passionate about youth development and arts and sports. She was also very involved with the Rotary Club in her town. And to Edie's father, her sister, and her, Ruth was the sun. Edie's father had even engraved "You are my sunshine" on the inside of Ruth's wedding ring.

When Ruth started to show concerning symptoms including balance issues, weight loss, nightmares, and sleeping difficulties, Edie called the doctor. By the time fall had changed to winter, Ruth's health had declined drastically. Then her symptoms became exacerbated after she fell and hit her head. Her voice went from a yell to a whisper, her short-term memory was nonexistent, and she developed a Parkinsonian tremor, but still, there were no answers to what was happening to her.

Edie took on the role of being Ruth's health advocate and chaperone. She drove her mother to her doctors' appointments while her sister did research, asked the hard questions, and sought clarity for an unknown diagnosis. Meanwhile, Edie's body spoke volumes to her; her intuition was screaming! Edie's knowledge and understanding of energy, body healing, and yes, even the corporate world all helped her as she stepped courageously into being Ruth's defender.

When Ruth was admitted to the hospital, Edie listened to the team of doctors tell them, "There are a few things she could have, one of which is Creutzfeldt-Jakob disease, but that's a one in a million chance, so don't worry, it's not that." But for Edie, she already knew in her gut that that was what her mother had. Weeks later, in the visitor lounge on the medical floor of the hospital, they had their confirmation. Ruth sat stoically as they told her that she was, indeed, one in a million and that her time was short.

Edie reached out to her therapist and received the most influential advice: "Tap into courage. Courage anchors you into your heart and into the moment, and you don't know how many moments you have left. When you want to run and shut down, lean in."

Edie shared this advice with her father and sister and understood the importance of her journey and of the day, a few months prior, when she stood with her palms open and said aloud, "Universe, I am ready to be of service."

Six weeks later, Ruth was admitted to hospice. Edie took on the heavy task of packing her mom's clothing and items to make her comfortable and at ease. And upon their arrival, Edie's first job was to decorate the room. She wanted to fill the space with joy, love, music, and dancing; she wanted to focus on living. As Edie began, she heard her mom whisper, "Edie, I want to go home." Edie whispered, "I love you, Mom" and walked out of the room to get some much-needed air.

As Ruth's energy declined and her systems began shutting down, the many people who had been impacted by her service wanted to see her and thank her for the life and legacy she'd lived. As Edie described it, Ruth was "sweet, appreciative, grateful for every visitor, the hospice staff—she was so kind, happy, and in grace."

Edie knew that she did not want to be in the room when her mother took her last breath. She felt that it would be the one moment she would not be able to handle. On the last night of her mother's life, Edie and her sister drove to the water to catch the sunset as a symbolic gesture of saying goodbye. It was as if the heavens had opened and the clouds became wings in the sky. A family of ducks made their procession into the water and for a moment, time stood still. Then the sky turned red, orange, and purple as the sun set over the escarpment.

Edie, her sister, and their dad spent that last night with Ruth. The next morning, Edie and her sister went home for some rest but received a call from their father within fifteen minutes. Ruth had taken her last breath. Together, Edie and her sister rushed back to their mother's room, and upon entering, saw their father holding their mother's hand while the song "Here Comes the Sun" played softly in the background. With deep sadness in his eyes, their dad said his last "I love you."

Edie was struck with a new understanding of life and death when she hugged her mother goodbye. Her body was limp, and Edie reflected that it is our soul that brings us to life, not our body.

Hundreds of people attended Ruth's celebration of life to share the memories they had of her. As Edie took it all in, she felt love, gratitude, and pride. One person can change everything and leave a mark on a community. This party was to honor Ruth's life as well as the people who were a part of it.

When the day came to resume their daily lives, Edie had new mantras dancing in her mind. She realized that we all make an impact in this experience called life, so we must love what we do and who we surround ourselves with; we must care for all people and not wait for the moment to be "right" to make changes.

She had heard the nudges, whispers, and callings before to focus on health and wellness, and now she was listening. Learning more about yoga, mindfulness, breath, and meditation became her focus. She became determined to bring a sense of belonging and community through the yoga practice to her world and to share with others the gifts of stillness and grounding found in meditation. These practices held Edie as she grieved, learned, and opened up to a space that her heart needed. It was finally time that Edie honored herself and her practice and fully believed in her own ability to leave a legacy.

YOURstory

Few things in life cause our heart to ache more than losing a loved one. In times of grief, we need to lean inward and carve out time for contemplation—about life, death, journeys, and healing. Through the grieving process, we need to ask ourselves what we need and want in life.

REFLECTION:

Diane Cooper, author and tarot card writer, wrote that "introspection is taking the time and the space for yourself to open up opportunities to recuperate from life's challenges, to reflect on the way ahead, strengthen yourself and prepare for the next phase of your life." Take a minute and find your center. What does your inner voice say to you? What are your needs, your wants? What do you desire?

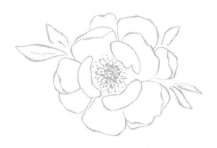

Chapter 11: Girl Time

I love winter! The coldest days bring out the brightest sunlight. The snowflakes sparkle and breathing in the fresh air can change any mood. I was banking on this happening as we moved into the new year with our shoulders up to our ears, still in stress mode from the holidays and all the changes we'd experienced with Sabrina's passing. My body didn't know how to release or unwind. My household didn't know how to function without an intense sense of urgency, fluctuating emotions, and an extra three bodies in it.

The six months since Sabrina's death had gone by in a blink, and everything had changed. Lillian and Everett didn't rely on me so much; it was as if they'd grown up and I missed it. I was slowly emerging back into life: I started seeing friends, engaging in social activities, and planning my tenth wedding anniversary with Darryl—a trip back to Dominica where we'd honeymooned. Our friends and family laughed when we told them, as there was an earthquake and tsunami warning during that honeymoon. But we had weathered storms before and planning the trip brought me joy and something to look forward to. I needed something happy to focus on—my connection with Darryl, the kids, and myself counted on it.

Upon our return home, I found myself feeling extremely exhausted and having severe headaches. My sleep was off, and my head was full of images, visions, and chatter. One day while the kids were at school, I decided to rest my head by taking a nap. Instead of sleeping, however, my daydream state was in overdrive.

Just over a year earlier at the November Evening Market & Bubbles party, I had mentioned to the crowd of ladies that I thought something bigger would come out of the events. Now, leaping from the bed, my energy spiked and my excitement vibrated. I had an idea that would bring change and be birthed out of what I had already created. A flood of information, visions, details, ideas, structures, and systems "downloaded" into my brain. I could see it all so clearly and knew that this idea was what I had been looking and asking for.

I had grown up watching my dad build a business from the ground up. I'd watched him work, talk shop, and put in the time, energy, money, and effort to create a business that he was proud of. I felt like I had all the education, life experience, drive, ambition, passion, and total grit it would take to start my own. I mapped it out and registered for free online business training, and I visited a group of entrepreneurs who got together weekly to learn from each other. I often woke up in the night with new ideas, content, mission/vision statements, and business models. I made numerous calls to business owners for advice. And in aligned timing at its finest, I met Aysia at a volunteer event. Aysia, a young website designer and marketing genius, was in charge of setting up all the web material for the committee running the event. We sat beside each other that day and had an instant connection. I knew she would be the first person I'd talk to about putting to life what had been keeping me up at night. My heart was leading the way.

Everything started to come into place and take form. One of the ladies Aysia was partnered with was a photographer who offered me a branding photoshoot package. I jumped at the opportunity. My vision was to showcase the different pillars of interest that Girl Time Inc. was going to offer to women. I had Lillian and Flinty join us on set. For Lillian, I wanted her there to see Mommy in action, to show her what following your dream looks like, and to be in a couple of the photos. As for Flinty, girl time is always better with a best friend beside you.

All the moving parts were flowing with ease and speed: the branding photos, the logo, and the slogan. Lillian and my nieces were my inspiration, as they were some of my biggest "whys" for creating the business. The whole idea of it evolved from wanting to build a company that would support HER. I was building a business that would focus on connection, the connection that I and so many women have longed for throughout our journeys.

At the heart of this longing came the unrealized WHY, the underlying current to create this business for women. In every chapter, every age and phase of my life, I had experienced the disconnect and isolation caused by sister wounds. Starting in childhood and following me all the way through to adulthood was the story that I was a threat to HER, to someone's competitive nature, to the constant judgment from comparison. Anytime I'd share my troubles, I'd hear comments like "They're just jealous; they're threatened by you" or "You are a lot; you're too much for them." I internalized these comments by believing that if I was "me," my real self, then I made other girls and women feel bad about themselves, that somehow it was my fault that they were threatened or didn't measure up. And inadvertently, that translated to "Be small to make others feel good about themselves."

Here I was, in creation mode of a business that would BE the space where women would feel safe, valued, heard, welcomed, and loved. Where they could BE all parts of themselves. I wanted it for me. Being the CEO and founder of Girl Time Inc. was like living in the shoes of my avatar. When everything around me was saying "live your best life," I took it literally and considered what that would mean for me. I had no idea what it would take to create the business, how much energy, time, and effort I would be expending, or what it would cost—both figuratively and literally. Nor did I realize what I would gain, how I would change, what would be exchanged for the better, or how much I would grow and heal. All I knew was that my heart was lit up. I was buzzing with ideas, plans, and people to connect, and I still had about a million steps to learn. But I had the confidence, grit, and courage to do it. Then, just as the pieces were lining up, COVID caused the world to stop.

I did not comprehend the level of energy, endurance, and true determination it was going to take to live through a global pandemic. Now, I'm typically not one to shut down when it comes to stressful times, but this was different. I was starting a business based on social activities, so that would have to change, something that made me nervous. But what I did know and could already see coming was that people would need connection. Feeling connected is what makes us human. I would have to make an adjustment to my plans to meet the significant need for connection, community, and collaboration to help women endure.

While thinking about my options, I had a sudden spark of inspiration. I knew I was not ready to launch the Girl Time Inc. platform just yet, but I also knew that I could create connection simply by being a voice. So I reached out to thirty women I knew and asked them if I could write a glimpse of their story. I would focus on how these women were leaders for us, our guiding lights.

I opened Girl Time Inc.'s Instagram account, and for thirty days I wrote these women's stories. I found inspirational quotes that matched HERstory and wrote about what she was actively doing to spark leadership, hope, and resilience. These "Featured Lady Posts" were received in love by an audience that was growing by the day, which brought me a newfound love for writing. In each post I wrote, I, too, was inspired by the women who showed up to share. Their stories had healing powers. I resonated with all of them and with every word I wrote, I let go and released into my own traumas and wounds.

My head was full of thoughts that kept me in forward motion, but I was not without limiting beliefs. One day while feeling the bigness of my vision, I became overwhelmed by insecurities and began to weep. My children, hearing me, ran to my side. They wiped away my tears with their tender touches and asked me why I was crying.

Long before they were born, I knew that when I became a mom, I would show my children all sides of me; I would show them my humanness. This was such a moment, one filled with vulnerability, fear, and insecurities mixed with courage and grit. To me, these are the best teachable moments. Fear showed up and with it all the conflict of holding on to my old life and the fear of what is to come with my new life. I explained that I was about to start a journey and create a dream that lived in my heart. I told them that it would require me to dedicate a ton of time, energy, and effort and that I would be working every day and into the night. I would be building a business from the ground up, just like my dad had, their papa. I held my babies tight and asked them for their permission to go on this journey. These were big concepts and big emotions for my children to witness. They gave me their blessing with kisses, hugs, and whispers that they believed in me.

I felt like a pioneer. A true trailblazer. I was inventing something that although not entirely new, seemed to be a new concept to many, mostly men. The businessmen that I was in contact with, the people who were going to help me build Girl Time Inc., were offering me good advice yet there was a disconnect. I was told multiple times that the business plan, structure, and model were too bold, too big, and that I would not be able to put it into action. There it was again—the outside voice, from an outside person, telling me that it was "too much," "I wasn't big enough to create it," and "the idea was too ambitious." Some women in business groups were no better. They, too, were wearing the masks of threat, comparison, and competition. It was like déjà vu. "Oh, you have so much energy." "You are always so happy and always put together."

"Aren't you just Little Miss Perfect." To my face or behind my back, I was getting my ass kicked by women throwing their dirty looks and energy blocks.

One businessman told me, "The vision is far too big, and you are not big enough to hold or create something of this caliber. It is a one in a million shot and not worth taking." I stood up, looked straight at him, and unapologetically said with a confident smile, "That is where we do not align. It is achievable. And you're wrong—it is one in a billion, but so am I." I walked away from that meeting feeling more encouraged than ever.

Girl Time Inc. was too advanced to be considered a "newbie," but it was not advanced enough to be considered expandable or ideal for growth. That left me in the gray zone. COVID was a hot mess everywhere. Everyone was pivoting their businesses, and some fell through the cracks of the helpful systems that had been put in place. I was one of them. The whole process felt frustrating. It was challenging for any new entrepreneur trying to find their way through it all.

Over a glass of wine with Darryl one night, I shared what was transpiring around me. Suddenly I had a flash of brilliance. I needed a team. I needed other women—boss women, leadership women, and badass women—who were taking on mountains just like I was. That night, I created Girl Time Inc. Ambassadorship. I knew who to call: women who needed me just as much as I needed them; women who would become the face of Girl Time Inc.'s pillars of interest. I pitched the idea. It would be a give-and-receive relationship and partnership that would bring our community of women the lift that they were craving: connection!

The first time I heard the word *Kula* was during an online yoga class with my favorite, heart-led instructor, Shirlee. She was speaking of the importance of community, and the word was like music to my ears. I researched it and then I pulled from it the roots to create a definition that Girl Time Inc. would be built on and grow from. Words matter. They hold magic and power! *Kula* was perfect and aligned deeply within me, so I trademarked it. It just made sense.

I'd established the pillars of Girl Time Inc., the foundation had taken shape, and I had my team. It was time to bring the calendar to life and into supersonic speed. COVID had created a sense of fear, and people needed hope, sparks of joy, and a sisterhood to show up; they needed leadership. My business advisers told me that it was time to switch into "green-light-go mode," so I did.

Together with Aysia, I shifted Girl Time Inc. from in-person events, socials, and activities to an online community. I reached out to other women entrepreneurs and told them that if we worked together in collaboration, we could create what I referred to as the infinity approach. I was creating a bridge between fabulous women in the community and fabulous women in business.

I had done this many times before with the Bubbles parties I had thrown. I knew what I was doing and was confident that it would work. We gained traction, and I put all my energy into getting ready for a June 1, 2020, launch and a full summer season. The world needed connection. Women in our area were searching for it. It was time to connect all the dots and find our Kula.

That first year was a rush. Having a heart-led business meant that when I was following the feeling, even directly into the unknown, I was doing so with the faith that no matter what, I was being guided. Anytime I switched directions to follow what someone else wanted me to do or I decided to go against my intuition, I got burned. So I did my best to stay true to myself.

The COVID world posed obstacles and hurdles that I had to figure out and maneuver. I sat in the front row of a roller coaster of successes and failures. To me, failure is an opportunity to grow, and that first year, I grew exponentially. I could plan only so far in advance. Although I was doing my best, there were so many times that my best was still not enough.

One day at a meeting with a fellow collaborator and friend, she asked me whether I was feeling burned out. I'd had a number of outside voices expressing the same: "You must be burned out." These comments fired me up. These people only had a glimpse of my world and of me. I was frustrated, but I knew my limits. I knew I wasn't burned out, but what exactly I was I had yet to discover. I was in a fog. I was having a hard time making decisions and coming up with ideas. I couldn't seem to figure anything out, and I didn't know where to start. I felt overwhelmed, confused, and lost.

As it turns out, a lot of people were feeling this way. There's actually a term for it: languishing. Adam Grant, in an article for the *New York Times* said, "Languishing is a sense of stagnation and emptiness. It feels as if you're muddling through your days, looking at your life through a foggy windshield. Languishing is the mid-man on the mental health spectrum. It sits right in between flourishing and depression."

It all made sense to me, and I could finally put a name to how I felt. Languishing had dulled my motivation and disrupted my ability to focus. To some degree, I knew what I was experiencing, yet I needed to let this feeling run its course. To the outside world, I was in a pink shirt and hustling. On the inside, I was fighting to find solid ground so I could pull myself to safety. I was not burned out, I was drowning in grief.

After a particularly heated meeting with my ambassadors one day, I snapped at my team. I was out of line and out of character. That morning, Everett had been crying about having to be on Zoom yet again. And Lillian, who was completely lost in school, was feeling the full effects of computer screen fatigue, so much so that her eyes were crossing. Darryl was on call, my friendships outside of my company were suffering and disappearing, and family issues were brought to the surface.

The stress of creating a calendar of events with socials and activities that supported the needs and wants of Girl Time Inc. members but stayed within the restricted lines of COVID regulations had done me in. I was not stressed or burned out; it was bigger than that. It was as if I'd opened Pandora's box. A massive storm of grief smacked me in the heart. A lifetime of old stories and flashbacks of sister wounds that had hurt me gushed out. I had been harboring these bruises for too long and I couldn't hold the weight and expectations of the job and business model plus what it asked of me the person.

When it rains it pours, as the saying goes. We had just listed our house for sale and we were searching for a new property. My shoulders could carry the load of everything, but the effects left me exhausted after every day. I knew that my capacity and capabilities were being tested. I was trying to regroup, but my fear, my feelings of inadequacy, put me in a panic. I had held it all together for well over a year, and as we were preparing to enter another season, everything got cloudy.

My light entered the room as I fell to my knees. Everett, the most empathetic person I know whose energy is pure love, and Lillian, my greatest teacher who is wise beyond her years, cradled me. Sitting in my own level of defeat, my babies found me yet again in my most vulnerable state. I explained that Mommy, who was trying to juggle all the different balls of life, had accidentally dropped a couple. Soft, loving voices soothed my wound: "Mommy, all messes can be cleaned up and all problems have solutions. You just have to try again and believe in your first step." One step is all it took. I stood, kissed their sweet cheeks, and cranked up the music. We danced, laughed, and sparked our joy. Music is a huge source of energy and motivation in our home. It has always been a tool I use to boost my mood and my sense of "go." I needed the perfect mix of music, movement, and love to shift my energy. From there, I would figure it out. I had to believe.

I started by owning up to my behavior and giving an apology to my team. I leaned on gratitude and thanked my friends and fellow boss ladies for holding me in integrity. I changed my mindset with the reminder and mantra "everything I need is already inside of me." I dropped the shield.

The second I surrendered to the process, let the light in, and asked for support, everything changed. Things shifted. The Girl Time Inc. social calendar came together brilliantly, and we had a season full of wonderful adventures. The team was united, lit up, and strong. My creative genes were back, and I saw visions for the future of Girl Time Inc. I saw details of a round table I would create and the book I was going to write. I was in full bloom.

My family life blossomed again as well. We sold our house and, in the search for a new one, divine intervention stepped in and took us back to the hamlet I'd grown up in, literally right to the property that my dad and grandfather once owned. The house needed some love and a makeover, but it was nothing I couldn't handle! And to add to our happiness, we added a Doberman pup to our household, something we had been talking about since my introduction to a "blue sky" life. And once the dust settled in my home and work life, I mapped out a road trip that would take me back throughout my own timeline and to the women who were a part of my journey.

That spring and into summer and fall, I went back to London, to Ottawa, to North Bay, to high school, to grade school, and then, to my family. I asked the women who were influential and legendary in my world to sit with me and share their wisdom, their stories, and our shared life journeys. I approached my antagonists—women who had betrayed our friendship, sold me out, and broken my heart. I sat in compassion, empathy, and love for them and for the story that we created together. I acknowledged my part in it all and how I'd, too, had a hand in their sister wound.

I sat in the living room of one woman who I hadn't seen since high school and apologized for the harm I did to her. I owned up to the pain I inflicted while releasing one of my darkest memories—the root cause. No more avoidance. I headed straight into my fears and came out the other side with more confidence, a clear definition of success, and a strong sense of self-love and sister love. Together, in the light and in the dark experiences, I understood that all these women were my greatest teachers.

My memories all connected—I understood the power of what I was creating and how to belong in true connection, in a Kula, and in sisterhood. I created a business that healed these wounds in every social, event, and activity I planned and participated in. It held power to create new opportunities to grow in love. Girl Time Inc. is my declaration of self-love. It's a validation not dependent upon other people but on my own self-worth and the power of it to get me through every journey I embark upon.

My stars were aligned, and my direction was upward and onward. My gratitude for the life I'd created was bigger than my feelings of languishing, words like *threat, comparison,* and *competition*, and all the old stories that hung in my closet. More than I'd like to admit, I've heard people say that I'm "too much." Now, for the first time ever, and right before I enter a new age and phase, I stand in that power and in the life that I've created for myself. I am no longer apologizing for being me. I am a magician, a queen bee and orca, a runner, a mother, a CEO and founder, a teammate and leader, and a partner and visionary who has big visions, dreams, and goals. And I needed to take on each of these titles (and so many more) to fully see what I am capable of and can do for HER—my daughter, my friends and family, women and girls, the audience I keep, my partners and collaborators, and most importantly, myself. I am capable of far more than I ever thought.

YOURstory

Successes and failures serve to teach us lessons. Success does not always come with a roar, but failure sure does sometimes. Outside voices and our own limiting beliefs can cripple us if we let them. But it is in these instances that we can find our strength. In these instances, we need to listen to our heart and the quiet voice that says, "I will try again."

REFLECTION:

Think of a time when your capacity and capabilities were tested. What gave you the motivation, inspiration, or push to get back on your feet?

Conclusion

When I began thinking about the idea for this book, I knew I'd be looking for a group of women who would be both brave and vulnerable and open and trusting in sharing stories of their female experience. Some women found me, while others were those I reached out to because they'd been influential women in my own journey. One such woman was Mia, a good friend of mine.

"Why me? There is nothing important about my story. What would I share?" she asked. Like so many women before her, she turned down the opportunity to share her story simply because she didn't recognize the value of it. As a witness to many of her amazing journeys, I realized then a new truth about women and life: until you shine a light on something, you don't necessarily see what has been there all along.

At the root of Mia's story is courage and determination to create a life for herself and her daughter that is bigger than the expectations and limitations placed on her. I remember sitting on her front porch and listening to her share about it:

"The hardest part was explaining to my father a year prior to my separation that my marriage was failing and that I didn't know what to do. I was seeking his advice, love, and support. Our conversation ended with his reply: 'You stay and stick it out—divorce is not an option.'"

Mia's story is one of high school love turned into loveless marriage built from convenience and societal pressures when they found out they were expecting. After years of disconnect, hardship, and fighting, Mia longed for something more. Then she received an "out" when her husband pointed to the door and told her to leave. So she did. She recognized the seriousness of her decision and what it would cost her financially, emotionally, and everything in between. Divorcing her husband meant much more than one failed relationship closing its doors: she was walking away from their friends and her own family who disapproved of her decision.

"I went from calling my mother multiple times a day to basically divorcing her too. The judgment and disappointment were unbearable for me to listen to. Why was something that felt so right to me so hard for everyone else? I was finally standing up for myself, believing that I deserved more. I was finally going after what I knew was right for me."

Mia broke the chain of societal expectations of women in her community the second she said she deserved better. Mia heard her inner voice, her self-worth speaking loud enough for her to choose the path less taken. She created a new home, found a new job, and made new friendships as a single mom. She became the heroine of her story, both for herself and for her daughter.

Mia's story represents a pattern: that "lightbulb moment" or the "last straw" is our inner voice reminding us of our self-worth. It is in all our stories and in every journey we go on. The second we hear it, believe in it, and step into it, we become our own heroes. Kristen, Vanessa, Barbara, Kristal, and all the ladies in this book, they all heard the voice and responded.

The Featured Lady Posts were the start of Girl Time Inc., the foundation that was built on the belief that when women see the importance of their self-worth and value, the community will rise up as a result. Women are searching for someone to hear, see, and value them, and to share women's stories is a way that other women can connect and feel that they are not alone.

Women's stories are important. And regardless of dark or light times, the female experience is universal. We've all experienced transitions and challenges, losses and heartache; we know what it's like to search out our identity and to find grit. We've all been "thrown from a horse" and had to stand up and brush ourselves off. We've all experienced defeat only to blossom again and again.

I was playing a game one night with a group of friends and was asked, "If you had a superpower, what would it be?" My answer was immediate. I have always wanted the ability to fly and have attempted flight many times. "Flight" to me came in the form of taking risks: hiking mountains in Switzerland, white-water rafting, skydiving, road and trail races, building a business that focuses on connection during COVID, and so on.

Now, upon looking back on my soon-to-be forty years of life, I would change my answer. The quote by Kurt Kaiser, "A bird sitting on a tree is never afraid of the branch breaking, because her trust is not on the branch but on her own wings," rings true to my heart. I realize that I already have a superpower: I am female. In every one of my stories, the victories and triumphs plus the failures and defeats, my superpower has appeared in my self-worth. No matter the severity of the dark or the brilliance of the light, my ability to love myself and to love others, and my own definition of success and my inner confidence, have all together made me mighty and powerful. The second we recognize our self-worth and how it gets us through each journey we face, we gain power. Once you tap into your own power, your self-worth, your importance, and what makes you sparkle, you tap into the magic of this life.

I am just at the beginning phases of writing HERstory and uncovering the strength, awareness, fearlessness, and empowerment of the female experience. Through sharing our stories and building this bridge, I hope that I will spark the individual that is you, unite the collective that is HER, and change the landscape that is for all of us. It's a new sisterhood. Our journey has just begun.

My bold, loving, and most sincere nudge is for you to recognize your worth, your inner confidence, your ability to love yourself and others, and your own definition of success. It is true: everything you will ever need is already in you. As for me, I'm at a new starting line. I have found my wings and I'm ready to fly.

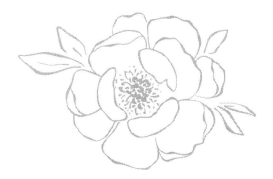

PS I am Barbara. xoxo

Acknowledgments

To express a genuine sense of gratitude is to notice and appreciate what is happening around you; to feel into the deep and personal experience and the positive chain of events and reactions. Focus, brighter, calmer—these are the chain reactions that happen in your mind. It is a wave of genuine gratitude, a physical and emotional connection with the body, mind, heart, and soul.

According to author and podcaster Mel Robbins, there are four essential elements to practicing genuine gratitude:

1. Specific: the "thing: experience, event, reaction" that triggers this form of profound gratitude
2. Deeply personal: it connects directly to YOU
3. WHY is it moving you? What is it about the "thing" that deeply and profoundly moves you?
4. The Feeling lingers (a lingering emotion)

The people in these acknowledgments have had a profound impact on my life and my story. To thank them is to actively practice genuine gratitude.

Darryl, you are my soul match. I would repeat every moment of our love story, both the light and dark parts. We have staying power. Some days I could just bite you, but god, you make me laugh. Thank you for going on this journey with me. You saw me at every stage of this writing process. Some moments were glorious, while others were a downright ugly hot mess with crying on our bedroom floor. You sat with me in both. You are my hero!

Lillian, I've wanted you my whole life. You are my dream come true. You were named after my favorite flower, the lily, and more specifically, the tiger lily. You are full of confidence, compassion, and virtue. You are a fierce young lady whom I admire for your independence, fiery determination, and sense of humor. I will do more than my best to be your guide, consultant, mother, and friend throughout the many rites of passage you go on as a female. Thank you for being my most powerful WHY—the why I do what I do for HER and that is you.

To my Everett, my anchor and my light. Wherever you are, there is love, playfulness, and adventure. You were my Mount Everest to climb, and upon reaching the top—you in my arms—my heart was complete as a mother. To love you is a gift that I will forever be grateful for. Along your journey, know that your superpower is your rainbow energy, pure love, compassion, and empathy. You have a hero's heart. Practice for greatness, Everett, and you will live the most magical life. Mommy loves you. Mommy loves you. Mommy loves you!

To both my children, I see you, I hear you, and I love you!

Bella, my black beauty and forever companion, thank you for keeping me company as I wrote. You always knew when to distract me and make me take breaks. Our walks cleared my mind or sparked new inspiration.

Meghan, Devon, Jen, and Crystal, thank you for being my forever friends. You have the other half of all my memories and stories. You know me to my very core and love me. You are the reason I know the love and joy one gets from an unbreakable sisterhood. You have always been my Kula and I love you for it.

To my girlfriends—you know who you are. You are the ladies who see all of me: the raw, real, let-my-hair-down me. My dancing partners, golf bitches, Halloween crew, and all the ladies who sit with me on my front porch and spend time with me! You are my soul sisters from Costa Rica, my running partners, and my hockey/dance mom friends! You fill my heart with joy, laughter, adventures, and fun. You are also the ones who I wrote about in the Introduction of this book. The women who have my heart. Thank you for being a huge part of my happiness and my memories!

To the Featured Ladies of *Writing HERstory*: Kristen, Morgan, Megan, Barbara, Alicia, Brittany, Cassandra, Marie, Rachel, Vanessa, Shannon, Lindsay, Annette, Samantha, Emily, Kristal, Magda, Edie, and Mia. Oh, ladies, you have changed my life. Sitting with you, listening, writing and being a witness to your stories has brought my life such purpose, strength, and great healing. I had no idea what I was creating at the beginning of this project and now, I am actively living into my self-worth. I see you—I see your journeys through the light and the dark and how the patterns that flow through each story align. I marvel at your grit, endurance, passion and compassion, self-love, and determination. You have inspired me to show up for my own story. Knowing that I stand with you gives me the courage to share my most sacred and vulnerable stories, the stories that make me who I am today. Thank you for trusting me with yours. Thank you for believing in me and going on a quest to write HERstory. I am honored, connected, and profoundly impacted.

To my mother, my sisters, and to all the women who have entered and exited my journey, antagonists or protagonists, you are my greatest teachers. Brief second to full season or lifetime, you have led me to where I am today, and for that I am grateful.

Dad, you are and will forever be my Superman. Thank you for sitting with me and being my sounding board, leader, and father. Thank you for showing me what grit is and to never give up on my dreams or myself. I learned the value of a handshake, the power of my word, and the importance of having integrity, a backbone, by watching you. Your balance of strength and softness is what I look up to and lean back on with full trust. I love you, Daddy!

To my brother Justin and sister Jayne, thank you for your friendship, support, and unconditional love. I know the love of sisterhood because of you, Jayne. Justin, you will forever be my first best friend. I can count on that, and I love you!

To Elaine and Al, my in-laws. You are my family in every sense of the word. Al, remember all the times you said, "No one remembers a good guy"? Well, maybe this time they will. Elaine, thank you for your love for and belief in me. Thank you for your unwavering support and how you love my children. It means the world to me, and I am beyond grateful.

To my soul sister in Heaven, Sabrina. Oh, girl, I miss you dearly! Thank you for seeing the vision of what is now here and alive in *Writing HERstory* and in Girl Time Inc. I can still hear your laughter, and when I see butterflies or dimes, I know it is you saying hello. Please know that I will forever honor my promise to you—it may be up close, near or far, but I will hold them forever in my purest sense of love. Thank you for trusting me with who you loved the most. Until we sip liquid salads again, I love you, my soul sister!

Thank you to all my teachers, mentors, principals, coaches, and run and yoga instructors for believing in me. Thank you for your knowledge, passion, expertise, and guidance. Thank you for challenging me to level up and tap into my own zones of genius. Your gentle pushes, little nudges, and time spent with me is appreciated and valued. Most importantly, thank you for seeing me and knowing that I had a sparkle and a light to shine.

To the Kula. You are influential and legendary women who celebrate inclusivity and a sense of belonging. You are also my healers. Your love, support, encouragement, and belief in me have set my soul free of the sister wounds that weighed on me. Thank you for your time—it is truly the most cherished gift you can give someone. Your spark of joy, happiness, health, and well-being will forever be my inspiration and dedication to Girl Time Inc.

To the Girl Time Inc. Ambassadors, all of you, thank you for seeing the vision, standing with me, and creating this space together. Mother Teresa's teachings captured the art and gift of collaboration when she wrote, "What I can do, you cannot. What you can do, I cannot. But together we can do something beautiful . . ." Oh, ladies! We sure did. Together, we have done something truly magnificent.

To Sabrina of YGTMedia, thank you for the nudge to find my inner writer. You saw what I did not know was possible. You saw the story in me. Your passion and heart-led leadership is changing lives, mine included. Thank you, Sabrina. xoxo

To Maya and Christine, my editors and team. Ladies, you made this experience a dream! Thank you for working beside me to make it a reality. I truly appreciate all the time, energy, and effort you put in. Your level of expertise, listening ability, and patience is so deeply valued. I thank you for seeing the vision, the big picture and ideas, and for helping me with the fine print. I would write a million HERstories with you as my team!

Last but not least, I want to thank myself! For the past two years, I have poured so much of my time, energy, love, and dedication into writing this book. I had no idea what it would take or ask of me to complete. Like all journeys, I started with a declaration that I was going to write not just my own story but also the stories of eighteen other women. I jumped in full-heartedly on a task that stretched, challenged, and built me like no other.

In writing the stories of the eighteen ladies, I started with an interview. These women came to my home where we sat for hours. They spoke, I wrote, and together, we healed. The most beautiful connections were made. They were deep with a full heart and vulnerability. It was the purest example of the healing powers that occur when women share their stories and actively support each other. We cracked open wounds and gave them a space to breathe, be seen, be valued, and be heard, and then, be told. I then took the time to sit in solitude and stillness to write HERstory. I tapped into HERstory, her energy, and wrote without second-guessing my words. I wrote from my heart, and like magic, HERstory was delivered along with my own.

This book is a mere glimpse of my life and some of the pinnacle moments that led me to where I am today. I am equally grateful for all my experiences, the connected dots. During this process, I worked through my own stories of sister wounds, heartaches, personal grief, insecurities, self-doubts, and childhood nightmares. I found unconditional love for my journey and became crystal clear on my definition of success, my ability to love myself and others, and on how strong my inner confidence truly is. My love for my story dissolved the hurt, the anger, and the separation I felt. For that alone, I am grateful for my courage to embark on this journey to my own self-worth. Journeys do that. They ask us to face our dark and honor our light with the hope that when we reach the other side, we learned the life lessons we needed to move into our futures. I can honestly say that writing this book did all of that for me.

I am also beyond words to describe the sense of gratitude I have for my soul's purpose. I had no idea what I was capable of but trusted that I could do it. And I did. Writing this book is by far the biggest gift to myself—to the eight-year-old version of me and to my future self. I have profound gratitude for my work ethic, dedication, discipline, grit, and writing abilities. I showed up for myself; I became my own hero.

Thank you, Miss Ashley!

Resources

If you are struggling with any of the challenges discussed in this book, the following organizations can offer support. Please note: These resources are specific to Canada. A quick Google search can help you find support and resources within your country.

ABUSE:
https://www.canada.ca/en/public-health/services/health-promotion/stop-family-violence/services.html

ADDICTION:
https://www.camh.ca/

EATING DISORDERS:
https://nedic.ca/

GRIEF AND BEREAVEMENT:
https://www.chpca.ca/resource/grief-and-bereavement-resource-repository/

POSTPARTUM SUPPORT INTERNATIONAL:
https://www.postpartum.net/

SEXUAL ASSAULT:
https://www.reescommunity.com/resources/

SUICIDAL IDEATION AND PREVENTION:
https://www.suicideinfo.ca/

References and Works Cited

BOOKS:

Morgan Harper Nichols. (2017) *Storyteller: 100 Poem Letters*. CreateSpace.

ARTICLES:

Simply Psychology. "Labeling Theory of Deviance in Sociology: Definitions & Examples" by Charolette Nickerson. May 10, 2023. https://www.simplypsychology.org/labeling-theory.html, accessed September 26, 2023.

The *New York Times*. "There's a Name for the Blah You're Feeling: It's Called Languishing" by Adam Grant. April 19, 2021. https://www.nytimes.com/2021/04/19/well/mind/covid-mental-health-languishing.html, accessed September 26, 2023.

WEBSITES:

https://www.postpartum.net/

VISUAL MEDIA:

Blake Edwards, dir. *Breakfast at Tiffany's*. Paramount, 1961.

Victor Fleming, dir. *Gone with the Wind*. Loew's Inc., 1939.

Darren Star, creator. *Beverly Hills, 90210*. Spelling Television, 1990–2000.

PODCAST:

Mel Robbins. The Mel Robbins Podcast. "The Science of Gratitude & 6 Surprising Ways You're Getting it Wrong." June 12, 2023. https://open.spotify.com/episode/5euE6Z2mu25lu4guwznNRq?si=DK_zt_O5S7Gm-mVPJJBfwCA

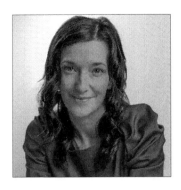

ASHLEY LOUGHEED is the CEO and founder of Girl Time Inc., a social club for women and women in business. Ashley's mission is to create a community—a Kula—for women, one where they can collaborate and create lifelong friendships, live a healthy and active lifestyle, and inspire each other to grow both individually and as a whole. She is the mother of two children, a newly published author, a public speaker, a leader, and a learner. Additionally, Ashley has a diverse education, including an honors degree in sociology, a bachelor of education, a degree in interior design, and a certificate in event planning.

Ashley believes wholeheartedly that it's time to connect and celebrate the rise of women as a collective vibration that is fueled with love and compassion, bravery and greatness, and empowerment and the readiness to thrive. She saw the needs, the wants, and the interests of women new and local to her town and has built a community to service those needs. At the end of the day, she is definitely a woman you want in your corner.

FOR MORE INFORMATION ON
GIRL TIME INC. AND WRITING HERSTORY, PLEASE VISIT:

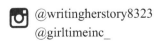 @writingherstory8323
@girltimeinc_

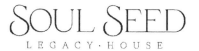

SOUL SEED
LEGACY · HOUSE

At Soul Seed Legacy House, we help thought leaders and creative entrepreneurs capture their vision in the form of nonfiction books, journals, workbooks, affirmation cards, and personal growth products.

Our mission is to help our authors grow and scale a platform far beyond the book, protect their soul's work, and turn their message into a legacy!

www.sslegacyhouse.com

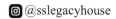 @sslegacyhouse

Manufactured by Amazon.ca
Bolton, ON